UNDERSTANDING CHRONIC FATIGUE SYNDROME

UNDERSTANDING CHRONIC FATIGUE SYNDROME

An Introduction for Patients and Caregivers

Naheed Ali

ROWMAN & LITTLEFIELD
Lanham • Boulder • New York • London

Published by Rowman & Littlefield
A wholly owned subsidiary of The Rowman & Littlefield Publishing Group,
Inc.
4501 Forbes Boulevard, Suite 200, Lanham, Maryland 20706
www.rowman.com

Unit A, Whitacre Mews, 26-34 Stannary Street, London SE11 4AB

British Library Cataloguing in Publication Information Available

Library of Congress Cataloging-in-Publication Data

Ali, Naheed, 1981-
Understanding chronic fatigue syndrome : an introduction for patients and caregivers / Naheed
Ali.
pages cm
Includes bibliographical references and index.
ISBN 978-1-4422-2657-9 (cloth : alk. paper) -- ISBN 978-1-4422-2658-6 (electronic)
1. Chronic fatigue syndrome--Popular works. 2. Caregivers--Popular works. I. Title.
RB150.F37A45 2015
616'.0478--dc23
2015011442

∞ ™ The paper used in this publication meets the minimum requirements of
American National Standard for Information Sciences Permanence of Paper
for Printed Library Materials, ANSI/NISO Z39.48-1992.

Printed in the United States of America

Understanding Chronic Fatigue Syndrome is dedicated to my readers, to chronic fatigue syndrome sufferers, and to all who provided encouragement and support for my research.

Also by Naheed Ali

Understanding Lung Cancer:
An Introduction for Patients and Caregivers

Understanding Celiac Disease:
An Introduction for Patients and Caregivers

Understanding Parkinson's Disease:
An Introduction for Patients and Caregivers

Understanding Alzheimer's:
An Introduction for Patients and Caregivers

The Obesity Reality:
A Comprehensive Approach to a Growing Problem

Arthritis and You:
A Comprehensive Digest for Patients and Caregivers

Diabetes and You:
A Comprehensive, Holistic Approach

Disclaimer

This book represents reference material only. It is not intended as a medical manual, and the data presented here are meant to assist the reader in making informed choices regarding wellness. This book is not a replacement for treatment(s) that the reader's personal physician may have suggested. If the reader believes he or she is experiencing a medical issue, professional medical help is recommended. Mention of particular products, companies, or authorities in this book does not entail endorsement by the publisher or author.

Author's Note

Understanding Chronic Fatigue Syndrome isn't meant entirely for medical professionals, yet the nonmedical reader may encounter advanced medical terminology. This is necessary to keep the book in line with the intended comprehensive review of chronic fatigue syndrome, and because certain medical concepts necessitate clarification well beyond a modest introduction. A glossary at the back of the book defines the complex lexicon to those who aren't familiar with the language of medicine.

CONTENTS

PREFACE

Chronic fatigue syndrome, otherwise known as CFS or myalgic en-cephalomyelitis (ME), is a complicated disorder that's primarily desig-nated by a feeling of severe exhaustion that doesn't get better with sleep or rest and that persists for at least six months.[1] Chronic fatigue syn-drome has also been called post-viral fatigue syndrome, chronic fatigue and immune dysfunction, as well as the "yuppie flu."[2] Severe exhaus-tion follows stressors such as physical activity and intense mental exer-tion.[3]

The syndrome can affect anyone—at any age and of either sex—but it's usually diagnosed in more women than men.[4] Likewise, it's seen in people who are obese or partake in a sedentary lifestyle.[5] Chronic fa-tigue syndrome affects about two out of every 1,000 individuals in the United States and about four of every 1,000 in the United Kingdom.[6] People who are diagnosed with chronic fatigue syndrome are said to have significantly lower activity levels when compared to the time be-fore they became unwell.[7]

Chronic fatigue syndrome can be described as mild, moderate, or severe.[8] Mild CFS involves difficulty or trouble doing simple tasks, but the individual is capable of moving as well as tending to necessities of life. Moderate CFS involves a termination of things that require labor or exertion, difficulty in sleeping, and moving around alone. Severe CFS embroils (a) the inability to do anything alone, (b) serious struggles regarding mental concentration, learning, and understanding, (c) the inability to move at all, and (d) sensitivity or irritability to noise and brightness.[9]

As of this writing, researchers have yet to identify a direct, significant cause of CFS or even a single test to diagnose CFS.[10] However, specialists theorize that chronic fatigue syndrome may be prompted by a combination of factors such as underlying medical conditions, infections, immune system problems, nutritional deficiencies, and stresses of psychological origin.[11] A series of tests may be needed to suitably diagnose chronic fatigue syndrome, as a number of other health conditions present matching symptoms that include sleep apnea, anemia, diabetes, insomnia, bipolar disorder, hypothyroidism, depression, and schizophrenia.[12] These tests take in full medical history and examination, mental status examination, full blood count (FBC), gluten sensitivity, erythrocyte sedimentation rate (ESR), creatinine kinase, and urine evaluation.[13]

Shared symptoms expressed by patients suffering from chronic fatigue syndrome include distended lymph nodes in the armpit or neck, persistent sore throat, muscle pain of unknown origin, unexplainable headache, severe feeling of exhaustion that continues for at least twenty-four hours following mental or physical stress, difficulty with memorization, joint pain, non-revitalizing rest or sleep, and, most importantly, fatigue.[14]

Before reading any further, the reader should understand that an individual is said to be suffering from chronic fatigue syndrome when he consistently experiences at least four of these symptoms for at least six months concurrently with, and not before, the fatigue itself.[15] Also, the fatigue shouldn't have been brought about or caused by in-progress physical or mental effort and the fatigue must impede simple everyday tasks. Other associated symptoms include chills and night sweats, allergies, irritable bowel, dizziness, fainting, balance problems or difficulty in standing up and maintaining proper posture, abdominal pain, panic attacks, chest pain, and shortness of breath.[16]

In general, the treatment for CFS is focused on relieving the symptoms, which can be accomplished by either medication or therapy.[17] Medications include antidepressant drugs that can partially alleviate or completely ease associated pain and sleeping pills that can help enhance sleep. Therapies include gradual physical exercise and psychological counseling.[18] In other cultures, especially Asian, one resorts to acupuncture, massage, yoga, or tai chi for symptom relief.[19] These methods are used to manage the symptoms but not to completely assuage the condition, so the most that they can do is to improve the quality of life of the individuals who have CFS. Unfortunately some clients don't fully recover.[20]

By now the reader might also wonder why CFS is a syndrome and not officially a disease. In reality, a condition, a term by which CFS is often correctly identified, is also classified as a syndrome when it's characterized by a set of symptoms occurring together, concurrently, and/or changing over time and when its cause is unknown.[21] On the other hand, a disease is present when the symptoms impair normal bodily function resulting in a sense of pain that has a proven source.[22] Since chronic fatigue syndrome is really a conglomerate of symptoms with no known cause, it's categorized as a syndrome and not a disease.

Moreover, a comprehensive approach to chronic fatigue syndrome, such as this book, is important, since individuals with chronic fatigue syndrome react to or handle the signs and symptoms differently; pain that's tolerable for one person could be debilitating for another, and depression brought about by the syndrome might be too much to take for an individual who doesn't know that he has CFS.

Needless to say, when this disorder is left ignored and unmanaged, it can be debilitating or incapacitating to the individuals who have it; it may significantly affect their livelihood as difficulty in moving, loss of concentration, social isolation, and depression become typical in un-compromising cases.[23] A comprehensive approach is also important since patients need to be aware of the real dangers of CFS—especially those who don't even realize that they suffer from it—so that it can be managed effectively, thus avoiding further possible complications.

Part I

Groundwork

I

ENERGY AND THE HUMAN BODY

Energy is defined as the exertion of power or the aptitude to do work.[1] Other definitions include the capacity to cause change and the ability to rearrange a collection of matter. In its different forms, energy can be kinetic energy or potential energy. Thermal energy, which implies movement of atoms or molecules, is kinetic in nature. However, chemical energy that's released in a chemical reaction is a form of potential energy.

BENEFITS OF HAVING ENERGY

Many unfortunate events are reported in the news every day, and for that reason, it's important to know that car accidents from drowsiness happen more frequently than those due to alcohol intoxication. In a recent survey, 27 percent of the participants admitted to dozing off at some point while they were driving.[2] That's because they lack energy to do their jobs properly and end up falling asleep at the wheel on their way home. There are also many reported suicide incidents caused by depression. That's in part because some people lack the energy to live when they face difficult challenges in their life. They become so hopeless that they resort to suicide as their way out.

The realities are alarming and these things happen mostly because of a lack of energy. Simple unfortunate events can also befall chronic fatigue syndrome (CFS) patients' daily lives. Some students taking im-

portant tests in school don't pass because they lack the energy to rumi-
nate answers correctly. They feel tired and reckon their minds aren't
functioning properly. Again, this happens because of lack of energy.[3]

The benefits of CFS patients having energy are virtually endless
because everything that they do requires energy. Without it, the examples mentioned earlier are just a few of the terrible scenarios that could
result at any time. These are some of the reasons why it's beneficial for
people to have bursts of energy. The good news for everyone is that
most accidents, failures, and calamities can be prevented with just a
simple rule: every person should have the energy to live gainfully, especially if these tasks are easy to do. Energy can be obtained by getting
ample sleep and consuming nutritious foods. There are simple benefits
of having energy. These advantages can be divided into three catego-
ries: physiological, occupational, and social and personal benefits.[4]

ENERGY AND METABOLISM

Energy in Relation to the CFS Patient's Body

Energy is necessary for learning and carrying out psychomotor skills
involving psychological processes associated with muscular movements
and the production of voluntary movements.[5] Examples of these skills
are running, swimming, jogging, bicycling, tennis, walking, golfing, driving a car, standing or sitting, and sleeping.[6] Energy buildup occurs by
increasing the intake of foods that are high in energy, by having adequate rest and sleep, and by treating pain.[7] Even when the CFS sufferer sits still, his heart continues to pump blood throughout his body.
Great amounts of food and energy aren't needed to keep it pumping,
but even so, more work requires more energy.[8]

Anyhow, the body uses some nutrients for energy. With it, a person
can move his muscles and be active. It helps him in repairing injuries to
his body. Whatever he does, nutrients serve up energy. Lastly, nutrients
are like the building provisions for a human body. They become a part
of the muscles, skin, bones, and other parts. Basically, they're essential
for growth.[9]

To conserve normal body functions (body temperature regulation,
muscular movement), the average person requires 2,000 to 3,000 calo-

ries per day. Calories in excess of what the CFS patient's body uses are stockpiled as fat, which then contributes to weight gain, whereas using more calories than are ingested fuels weight loss. As a general rule, 3,500 calories are equivalent to approximately a pound of body weight. Certain activities burn body weight to yield energy such as running, which has an energy output of 0.110 calories per minute, per pound of body weight.[10]

ENERGY AND THE NERVOUS AND ENDOCRINE SYSTEMS

Since neurologists often see chronic fatigue syndrome patients, it's prudent for the reader to understand how energy plays a role in the nervous and endocrine systems.

The Nervous System's Role in Energy Production

Cerebrospinal fluid formed in the brain by filtration of blood circulates slowly through the central canal and ventricles of the brain and then drains into the veins, assisting in the delivery of nutrients and hormones to unique regions of the brain and in the removal of waste. This is one way in which the CFS patient garners energy.[11]

Sensory neurons send information about the internal and external environment to the brain while the motor neurons control the muscles and glands. Brain cells connect the motor and sensory pathways, monitor body processes, take action on the internal and external stimuli, maintain *homeostasis*, and orchestrate psychological, biological, and physical activities.[12]

The Endocrine System's Role in Energy Production

The endocrine system is the interconnected network of glands. Due to its links to the nervous system and the immune system, the endocrine system has far-reaching energy-producing effects in the chronic fatigue syndrome patient. The hormones emitted by this system are affected greatly by organs such as the hypothalamus. Other structures in the brain, some of which are endocrine system glands, also manipulate the function of other endocrine glands. The energy-providing hormones secreted by the endocrine system affect the nervous system, but at times, the latter system also intervenes. For example, norepinephrine and epinephrine, which are secreted by the adrenal medulla, act as neurotransmitters.

ENERGY AND THE RESPIRATORY AND CIRCULATORY SYSTEMS

The upper and lower respiratory tracts constitute the respiratory system. Together, the two tracts are responsible for ventilation, the movement of air in and out of the airways. The upper respiratory tract, also known as the upper airway, warms and filters air so that the lower respiratory tract, the lungs, can accomplish gas exchange. The process of gas exchange involves delivering oxygen to the tissues through the bloodstream and expelling waste gases such as carbon dioxide during expiration. The respiratory system works together with the circulatory system. The former is accountable for ventilation and diffusion while the circulatory system is responsible for *perfusion*.[13]

Breathing Control and Energy

Humans can voluntarily hold their breath, but most of the time, automatic nervous mechanisms oversee breathing. Without inhalation, individuals with CFS wouldn't have any energy at all. This ensures that the work of the respiratory system is coordinated with that of the heart and with metabolic demands for oxygen. The main breathing control centers are located in two regions of the brain, the medulla oblongata and the pons.[14]

Breathing control is effective only if it's coordinated with control of the cardiovascular system so that there's a good match between lung ventilation and the amount of blood flowing through the alveolar capillaries. For instance, during exercise, increased cardiac output is matched to the increased breathing rate that enhances oxygen uptake and carbon dioxide removal as blood traverses through the lungs. By extension, this is how the CFS patient's body regulates its own energy.[15]

ENERGY AND THE MUSCULOSKELETAL AND DIGESTIVE SYSTEMS

The musculoskeletal system includes the bones, joints, muscles, tendons, ligaments, and *bursae*. These components function in an integrated manner. The health and proper functioning of this system is interdependent with that of the other body systems. The system, which is fundamental for the use and buildup of energy, also (a) provides protection for vital organs, including the brain, heart, and lungs, and (b) offers a resilient framework to support body structures. It makes moving possible.[16]

ANALYSIS

All of the cells of the body require nutrients, and energy production is the denouement. Without energy, CFS patients can't carry out daily functions properly. Food that contains proteins, fats, carbohydrates, vitamins, minerals, and cellulose fibers and other vegetable matter is the birthplace of these nutrients and therefore serves as the foundation of energy for the CFS sufferer.

There's no dependable formula for simultaneously attaining happiness and satisfaction, enjoying a long life, getting a job promotion, or becoming famous. Nonetheless, if a CFS patient has adequate energy for everything he does, he'll get more or less all of the benefit there is to receive in the physiological, occupational, personal, and social aspects of his life.

2

HISTORY OF CHRONIC FATIGUE SYNDROME

In recent years, chronic fatigue syndrome (CFS) has been popularized as an illness of the twentieth century. However, the disorder isn't entirely novel. In fact, there are a number of reports of diseases similar to chronic fatigue syndrome dating back as early as two hundred years ago.[1]

EVOLUTION OF THE TERM "CHRONIC FATIGUE SYNDROME"

The long history of CFS has been surrounded by rightful controversy in both defining and naming it. Naming a disease such as CFS imposes a great challenge because the selected name can influence how the patients are perceived and treated by society, including by those involved in their treatment and their families, friends, and coworkers. Since its discovery, the syndrome has undergone many name changes before a trove of scientists coined the name "chronic fatigue syndrome" in 1988. Even in recent years, its name is controversial.[2]

Febricula and Neurasthenia

In 1750, Sir Richard Manningham reported a syndrome that was known as *febricula*, otherwise called little fever, a disease characterized by a

copious number of symptoms that were difficult to diagnose objective-
ly.[3] In the nineteenth century, an American psychiatrist and neurologist, George Miller Beard, popularized the concept of *neurasthenia*.
This disease was thought to be nervous system mayhem characterized
by enfeeblement of nerve forces.[4] Fatigue, anxiety, headache, and im-
potence, as well as neuralgia and depression, were among neurasthenia's reported symptoms.[5] It seemed that young women were more
susceptible to the disease and its onset was most often triggered by an
infection.[6] Lasting tiredness was seen as the primary symptom with the
cardinal sign being an inordinate sense of physical or mental fatigue.[7]

One of the most famous historical figures who might have been
victimized by CFS was Florence Nightingale, known as the mother of
modern nursing.[8] In fact, Nightingale's birthday (May 12) is International ME/CFS and Fibromyalgia Day. It was reported that her illness
started after returning from the Crimean War, when she spent years
lying on a bed too exhausted to talk to more than one visitor at a time.[9]

She suffered from obdurate pain and fatigue for a large part of her
life. Fascinatingly, shortly after her death, medical opinion favored the
idea that she'd been suffering from neurasthenia. The concept of neurasthenia was actually commercialized by Beard in the 1880s, who described the illness prevalent among young women with a great resem-
blance to the disease that's now embedded in medicine as fibromyalgia.[10]

The censures of neurasthenia involved widespread pain, fatigue, dizziness, palpitations, and psychological problems. Neurasthenia, in fact,
literally means "nervous exhaustion." The wide gamut of symptoms experienced by Florence Nightingale led to speculation that she suffered
from CFS, fibromyalgia, or even post-traumatic stress disorder. Others
refuted this view and claimed that Florence Nightingale was suffering
from brucellosis, a chronic bacterial infection with nonspecific symptoms.[11]

Although it's difficult to ascertain an accurate diagnosis for Nightingale's condition, research suggests that bacterial or viral infections are
risk factors for the development of chronic fatigue syndrome. Furthermore, recent findings assert that chronic bacterial infection may in fact
be a cause of CFS.[12]

In current times, neurasthenia is perceived as a behavioral rather
than a physical condition. However, it isn't considered a medical diag-

nosis.[13] As of this time, the World Health Organization's ICD-10 system categorizes neurasthenia under category F48 ("other neurotic disorders"), which specifically excludes chronic fatigue syndrome. As neurasthenia began to lose popularity, two episodes of CFS, which involved doctors and nursing staff, occurred in successive decades and grabbed hold of the public's attention. These outbreaks also gave rise to various names for CFS.[14]

Poliomyelitis

The first-ever recorded outbreak of CFS known widely occurred at the Los Angeles County General Hospital in 1934. Symptoms included muscle pain of long duration, tenderness, weakness, and sensory symptoms, lapses in memory, difficulty in concentration, sleep disturbance, instability of emotions, and inability to walk short distances without suffering fatigue. Around two hundred members of the hospital staff acquired the disorder, due to which more than half of them were still unable to work six months later.[15] Initially, it was thought the unknown illness might be related to polio. However, the patients' muscles didn't waste away as they did with polio. This all subsequently provided a scrupulous explanation of what unfolds in a CFS patient's organs.

Similar outbreaks of the disease initially thought of as poliomyelitis also underwrote the long history of the syndrome before it finally came to be known as chronic fatigue syndrome. At a Wisconsin convent, apprentices and administration candidates were detected with a disease that they called encephalitis in 1936. In 1937, two towns in Switzerland had outbreaks of "abortive poliomyelitis." Two years later, more than seventy Swiss soldiers were diagnosed with the same.[16] In 1938, Alexander Gilliam reviewed medical records and interviewed patients affected by the outbreak in Los Angeles Country General Hospital. Gilliam referred to the disorder that infected staff as "atypical poliomyelitis."[17]

Iceland Disease

More than a decade since the Los Angeles epidemic, an outbreak of a disorder very similar to poliomyelitis occurred in Akureyri in northern Iceland.[18] That explains why CFS is also called Akureyri disease or Iceland disease. The first case of the outbreak was reported in Iceland on September 25, 1948. The spate of disease there affected more than 1,000 people. Interestingly, a successive polio epidemic on the island in 1955 didn't affect the town. Speculators then argued that the virus, which may have caused the CFS outbreak, resulted in providing a level of immunity to polio.[19]

The main clinical offshoots were tiredness and exhaustion and the disorder was still diagnosed as poliomyelitis. Between the third and fourth weeks of November, the outbreak was differentiated from epidemics of poliomyelitis. It lasted for more than three months and yielded hundreds of reported cases.[20]

Royal Free Disease

Miniature outbreaks occurred in the United Kingdom: Middlesex in 1952, Newscastle in 1959, and London from 1970 to 1971. The number of cases recorded reached 150. As a result, the United Kingdom, together with the United States, is now arguably at the crest of CFS research.[21] In late spring of 1955, an outbreak occurred at the Royal Free Hospital, probably the most well-known incidence of chronic fatigue syndrome on a large scale in the United Kingdom. The incident, which commenced when the hospital admitted a number of people with bizarre symptoms, lasted more than four and a half months. Events drastically unfolded when in July of the same year, around 300 staff members fell ill, of whom 255 needed to be quarantined on hospital grounds. To this end, the hospital was forced to go bust in the early part of October.[22]

Interestingly, only 12 percent of the nearly 300 people affected were in-hospital subjects at the time of the epidemic. Symptoms developed initially from a flu-like malaise that later became more prominent after a short remission, with a new group of symptoms arising. The most noticeable clinical sign of the disorder was extreme muscle fatigue after minimal exertion. Other symptoms were related to brain function, specifically with short-term memory and concentration. Headaches, blurred vision, and unusual skin sensations were also reported as indications. The medical examination conducted afterward concluded that roughly 70 percent of the patients had their central nervous systems bungled by CFS.[23]

The disorder now known as chronic fatigue syndrome was later coined by Melvin Ramsay, who was the medical consultant in charge at the time. Based on this outbreak, "myalgic encephalomyelitis" was defined by Donald Acheson in an editorial entitled *A New Clinical Entity?* that was published in *The Lancet* in 1956. Acheson named the disorder "benign myalgic encephalomyelitis," with *benign* denoting a zero mortality rate.[24]

The article covered selected epidemic outbreaks that happened in the years prior, according to the description of Ramsay and others. In 1981, Ramsay finally published his designation of the disease, naming it myalgic encephalomyelitis. The definition included four central tenets: (1) fatigue after minimal exertion and delay of recovery of muscle power after exertion ends, (2) one or more symptoms indicating circulatory impairment, (3) one or more symptoms indicating involvement of the central nervous system, and (4) wavering symptoms.[25]

Tapanui Flu

In Australia, one of the earliest occurrences of CFS happened in Adelaide in 1949. Hundreds of unwitting patients were confined to the hospital due to a CFS-like infirmity. Australia had also been piloting research on CFS, especially in regard to immunology, infection, and management. In 1998, they created a working group that provided instructions to best diagnose and manage people with CFS.[26]

Chronic fatigue syndrome disembarked on the South Island region of Otago, New Zealand, in 1984. Due to the location of the outbreak, CFS was dubbed the Tapanui flu. The patients initially developed a flu-like malaise and suffered from fatigue that incapacitated them for several weeks. A ten-year study was conducted following the outbreak on twenty-one of the patients who were affected. The journal *Archives of Internal Medicine* reported that sixteen of twenty-one victims who had the illness achieved a nearly perfect degree of functioning by the culmination of the ten-year period.[27]

Epstein-Barr and the Yuppie Flu

In 1984, another similar outbreak unraveled in the Lake Tahoe locale of Nevada, which caught significant attention from the U.S. public and media. In the latter part of 1984 a number of healthy adults suddenly displayed symptoms of an unusual flulike affliction followed by symptoms related to myalgic encephalomyelitis or chronic fatigue syndrome, namely, muscular fatigue and cognitive degeneration. Doctors examining the patients affected were skeptical about whether the latter were physically ill since blood tests failed to bring anything unusual to light.[28]

Around that time, researchers started to ponder whether the disorder was related to the Epstein-Barr virus (the virus linked with gland-based fever) or infectious mononucleosis. However, clinical research findings demonstrated that even though three-quarters of the patients had high levels of Epstein-Barr virus antibodies, the rest had no virus or no E-B virus antibodies at all. Their theory also appeared questionable because E-B virus antibody tests were difficult to deduce. The various test results were highly similar to the anticipated results from normal, healthy adults coming from similar backgrounds. In addition, by age thirty, most people had been exposed to the E-B virus with only a selected few developing glandular fever.[29]

Despite the incongruence, CFS grew in popularity as the U.S. media publicized it unsparingly. *Newsweek* labeled it the malaise of the '80s. Others called it "yuppie flu" because most of the affected population were young and active professionals. Although its relationship with glandular fever virus was also uncertain, it seemed that the public's curiosity about the disorder was satiated with the new aliases they had given it: chronic Epstein-Barr virus (CEBV) or chronic mononucleosis. These two terms became widely accepted.[30]

Another trendy U.S. magazine, *Hippocrates*, publicized the epidemic at Lake Tahoe when it published an issue with a cover story about the epidemic. However, despite its established title—CEBV—the magazine used another name—Raggedy Ann syndrome—to reflect the fatigue and loss of muscle power experienced by the patients.[31]

The National Institute of Allergy and Infectious Diseases held a consensus conference in 1985 when chronic Epstein-Barr virus or CEBV was used to describe the CFS-like symptoms. CEBV became the well-known term for the disorder at that time, and academic journals considered it a legitimate medical disorder. In 1987, two years after chronic Epstein-Barr virus gained popularity as the name of choice for the disorder, the CEBV Association was established by Mark Iverson and Alan Goldberg.[32]

The group's name was later on changed to the CFIDS Association of America. This was the suggestion of Seymour Grufferman, an immunologist who recommended the name "chronic fatigue immune dysfunction syndrome" in order to reflect more on the immune anomalies of the condition rather than fatigue as the prominent symptom.[33]

Issues with Nomenclature

In 1988, researchers primarily from the Centers for Disease Prevention, or CDC, coined the term *chronic fatigue syndrome* to describe the most prominent symptom of the illness. A new case definition was also developed using the Holmes criteria.[34] Other "medical-sounding" terms were also suggested but dismissed due to the lack of definitive evidence of a causative agent. Even though the syndrome was finally called by a name that's most appropriate for it, the naming of CFS still didn't come easy, as issues continue to surface from time to time.

In 1996, Kenneth Calman, then the United Kingdom's chief medical officer (CMO), requested a commentary from the Royal Colleges of Physicians, Psychiatrists, and General Practitioners. This soon led to the release of a report supporting that "chronic fatigue syndrome" was found to be the most fitting term. This was further supported by a follow-up report in 2002 by Liam Donaldson, the new CMO.[35]

However, CFS terminology still remains highly divisive.[36] There are a remarkably high percentage of patients affected by this illness who have received disrespect and poor treatment by the medical world. The name of an illness, therefore, is very important in how it's perceived by the general populace. It's essential to know and review the issues concerning the terminology of CFS to understand the public's cynicism and stigma toward the patients.

Although the term *chronic fatigue syndrome* was chosen because fatigue was considered the apex symptom of the illness in question, the new phrase received only negative feedback from the patients.[37] They believe that naming the disorder CFS belittled its seriousness. This is due to the fact that the illness is typified by many severe symptoms aside from fatigue. Fatigue is also a common symptom in the general population, even for healthy individuals.[38]

In 2001 and 2002, two consecutive studies were announced to determine whether the alternative names of CFS—chronic fatigue syndrome and myalgic encephalopathy—affected the academic efforts of college undergraduates and medical trainees concerning the syndrome.[39] Participants were randomly divided into two groups, each with different diagnostic labels used in a case description of a patient with symptoms of chronic fatigue syndrome. The studies concluded that the characteristics that participants attributed to CFS depended on the different diagnostic labels used to characterize it. The results showed that the diagnostic name myalgic encephalopathy (ME) paralleled the worse prognosis.[40]

Myalgic encephalopathy was also more likely to be linked with a physiological rather than psychosocial origin, thus requiring nonpsychiatric treatment when compared with those with the title "CFS."[41] A high number of patients believed that changing the name from myalgic encephalomyelitis to chronic fatigue syndrome was a major contributing factor to the stigma this disorder received.

Due to these issues surrounding CFS, there have been continual studies regarding its name. During the summer of 2000, the CFS Coordinating Committee (CFSCC) of the Department of Health and Human Services appointed a name change workgroup (NCW). The group aimed to change the name from "chronic fatigue syndrome" to one that perfectly reflected the severity of the syndrome and the organ systems affected.[42]

One alternative that NCW considered was NEID, or neuro-endocrine immune disorder, due to the growing scientific evidence of neurological, neuroendocrine, and immune system dysfunctions in patients shaken by this syndrome. Myalgic encephalomyelitis or myalgic encephalopathy was also suggested as an official label for the syndrome, considering that myalgic encephalomyelitis had been used prior to the term CFS. According to a study in 2001, most of the roughly 430 respondents (85 percent) indicated that they wanted a name change. However, both the patients and the physicians were split between adopting a name such as myalgic encephalopathy (ME) or one such as neuro-endocrine immune disorder (NEID). The survey also indicated that the acronym NEID had certain pejorative characteristics. Thus the NCW members were compelled to think of a better name for the syndrome.[43]

Since the results of the studies showed that the previous labels for the syndrome weren't the preferred choices, the NCW negotiated the umbrella term "chronic neuroendocrine immune syndrome," or CNDS, under which patients could be classified into subgroups according to their symptoms and pathophysiology.[44]

One of these subgroups would be myalgic encepahalomyelitis or myalgic encephalopathy. This recommendation was based on (a) the frequency of the reported symptoms of patients with the syndrome, (b) chronicity of the illness, (c) the lack of an understanding of its causes, and (d) insufficient published evidence supporting an abnormality in the neurologic, endocrine, and immune systems. In 2002, researchers facilitated two surveys that found that between 57 and 66 percent of patients and health care providers endorsed the term CNDS.[45]

Still, there are CFS experts who argue that the current name still factors in the invalidation and stigmatization of the disease. Due to the controversy revolving around the name and diagnosis of CFS, patients affected with the syndrome face skeptical attitudes, and many of them suffer great losses in their support system.[46]

CHRONIC FATIGUE SYNDROME AND FAME

Celebrities are no exception to the far-reaching outcomes of CFS. Here is a synopsis of celebrities who have been known to battle this syndrome.

Michelle Akers

Born February 1, 1966, in Santa Clara, California, Michelle A. Akers is a former American soccer star despite her long-term battle against chronic fatigue syndrome. She was born to Robert and Anne Akers and grew up in a suburb in Seattle, Washington, where she attended and played soccer for Shorecrest High School. She was dubbed an All-American three times during her high school career. After her retirement, she continued to promote the game of soccer. One of her books chronicled her battle with chronic fatigue syndrome, the disorder that hampered her training during the last eight years of her career.[47]

Susan Blackmore

A renowned figure in England, Susan Blackmore is the author and contributor of more than sixty academic articles and forty books.[48] She's also famous for her book *The Meme Machine*. Aside from being a writer, Susan is a lecturer, skeptic, and broadcaster on psychology and the paranormal. She's a contributor to *The Guardian* newspaper, and she earned degrees in psychology and physiology from Oxford University and a PhD degree in parapsychology from the University of Surrey. She spent decades proving to her colleagues at Oxford that the paranormal does exist. Afterward, she changed her beliefs, which was considered a devastating blow to her, ultimately turning her identity upside down.[49]

In 1995, she developed CFS after spending many long hours on different projects. She couldn't manage to walk and couldn't bring herself to a relaxing sleep. Reading and concentrating were also difficult for her, except for short periods. The syndrome, however, became a positive aspect of her life as it led to her discovery of a new branch of science: cultural evolution, or memes, in which humans store ideas, art, stories, technologies, and science and pass them to the next generation, just like that seen in genetics. Thankfully, CFS gave her a whole new perspective on life.[50]

Cher

Cher is an American singer and actress and one of the world's most celebrated stars. Born May 20, 1946, as Cherilyn Sarkisian in El Centro, California, Cher was nicknamed the "goddess of pop." Cher has proven herself to be a consummate entertainer with platinum-selling albums, sold-out concerts, award-winning movies, and famed television shows. Cher started her career as half of a singing act with her then-husband Sonny Bono in the 1960s.[51]

In the 1990s, Cher suffered from chronic fatigue syndrome for three years. She developed bronchitis and pneumonia because of CFS. During this period, she had to drag herself to her performances and occasionally cancel her shows. In an interview in 1999, she told Larry King that no one believed her for a long time. Traditional doctors didn't have a clue as to what she was suffering from. It was only when a homeopathic physician believed her complaints and sympathized with her that she finally made her way to recovery.[52]

Blake Edwards

Born as William Blake Crump in July 26, 1922, Edwards was an American film director, screenwriter and producer. Edwards started off as an actor in the 1940s, but his interest in acting soon waned, and he turned to screenplays and radio scripts and then to producing and directing film and TV shows. His most famous films are *Breakfast at Tiffany's*, *Days of Wine and Roses*, and the hit *Pink Panther*.[53]

He was famous for directing comedies, but he also directed other film genres, such as drama and mystery. Although he suffered from CFS for years, he was able to find ways to continue his career. Edwards died in December 15, 2010, at eighty-eight due to pneumonia.[54]

Amy Peterson

Amy Peterson is an American short-track speed skater who competed in five consecutive Olympic Games, from the time that short-track speed skating was an exhibition sport in 1988 until 2002.[55] Peterson was only in her teens when she qualified for her first Olympics in 1988 in Calgary.[56] She had an ongoing battle against CFS, which eventually ended her participation in the Olympics. She returned to qualify for the Winter Olympics in Japan in 1998 after overcoming the syndrome. Peterson's career suffered at that time with her Olympic rankings tumbling.[57]

Stevie Nicks

Stephanie "Stevie" Nicks, a well-known American singer and songwriter, produced more than forty top-fifty hits and unloaded more than 140 million in album sales. She was considered the "reigning queen of rock and roll" as well as one of the 100 greatest singers of all time.[58] In 1998, she was inducted into the Rock and Roll Hall of Fame. She also has won a total of eight Grammy Award nominations as a solo artist.[59]

Around 1986, Nicks developed an addiction to cocaine, which her doctor warned could lead to severe health problems. Although her cocaine consumption didn't directly lead to her CFS, in 1987, one of Nicks's tours was suspended due to her symptoms of chronic fatigue syndrome and slowly developing addiction to clonazepam. Nicks was still able to pull through with great career in the entertainment business in the following year.[60]

ANALYSIS

The reason that chronic fatigue syndrome has gained the image of a new disorder can be traced to its long history of having various titles, leading it to be labeled as the disease of a thousand names.[61] A thousand may be an exaggeration, but there's indeed a long list of names that were used for this disorder in different parts of the world and during different eras.

Part II

Clinical Picture

3

CAUSES AND RISK FACTORS

Although chronic fatigue syndrome (CFS) isn't a new medical discovery, its causes remain unknown today. Scientists and researchers have yet to determine a precise explanation for what triggers CFS due to the heterogeneous and inconsistent symptoms present in patients diagnosed with the disorder.

SUSPECTED CAUSES

Patients with CFS have reported that they had experienced moderate to severe physical pain (possibly caused by viral infections) or emotional instability involving depression before developing CFS. These symptoms, whether alone or combined, have led medical experts to believe that the nervous system and a gene abnormality could possibly trigger CFS. However, medical experts haven't discovered a specific brain or nervous system hindrance that's consistent in every patient.[1]

Continuing studies are still in progress. As of late, only logged medical theories can provide information about the supposed sources of CFS. The symptoms listed in these medical theories have been observed to be the most common similarities among patients diagnosed with chronic fatigue syndrome. Medical speculations that attempt to resolve the causes of CFS state the following probable reasons: viral infection, genes, brain defects, an overreactive immune system, psychiatric or emotional conditions, and stress-related hormonal abnormalities. These are some of the more prevalent theories involving the grounds of CFS.[2]

Viral Infections

Researchers believe that a viral infection may cause CFS because its symptoms are similar to that of an infection. Sadly, this claim is idiosyncratic since not all patients with CFS have had a serious infection. This led researchers to consider that there may be two causes of CFS: viral and nonviral causes. Medical studies haven't discovered a single viral infection that may have a direct relation with CFS even though these infections share the same symptoms with CFS. Some of the viruses that have been scrutinized include the following:[3]

- Epstein-Barr virus infection, otherwise known as mononucleosis;
- Human herpesvirus 6 infections, which is problematic for those with impaired immune systems;
- Enterovirus infection, a type of virus found in the gastrointestinal tract that isn't severe or deadly. This form of infection shows mild flu-like symptoms;
- Rubella, more commonly known as German measles;
- *Candida albicans*, a type of fungus that can cause yeast infections;
- Borna viruses, known to cause the infectious Borna disease;
- Mycoplasma, which causes atypical pneumonia;
- Ross River virus, a virus that begets Ross River fever, a mosquito-borne tropical illness;
- *Coxiellaburnetti*, the infectious agent that caused Q fever; and
- Human retrovirus infection, such as HIV or xenotropic murine leukemia virus-related virus (XMRV), a gamma retrovirus.

A study states that patients who have had stark viral septicity are more likely to be diagnosed with CFS than other patients, which leads medical pundits to believe there may be more than one way to contract CFS.

Genetics

According to various clinical investigations, genetics may be a possible culprit lurking in the shadows of CFS.[4] These studies show that there are certain genetic characteristics that may put some patients at more risk than others. Researchers affirm that genes that are linked to infections and blood disease may cause CFS. Furthermore, genes overseeing the body's response to stressful and traumatic injuries may also be a contributing factor of CFS.[5]

Genetic components involved in the functions of the immune system, communication between cells, and the transfer of energy to cells are also listed as a possible cause. Many medical findings have indicated that a patient's immune system may lead to CFS. Unfortunately, despite studies claiming that viral infections may be a direct cause, a patient's immune system isn't the sole basis of CFS. Since the syndrome is held to have been brought about by viral infections, medical experts theorized that genetic predisposition could only exacerbate the development of CFS in a human being.[6]

When a patient encounters a viral infection, his body generates cytokines. Cytokines are a group of proteins relinquished by certain cells in the immune system.[7] Chronic fatigue syndrome patients have exhibited, possibly genetically, a significantly elevated level of circulating cytokines.[8] Antibodies in the immune system are proved to be positive among CFS patients, but again, there hasn't been a direct genetic link that would lead researchers to believe that such circumstances lead to the disorder.

No typical tissue disconcertion related to autoimmune disease has been indicated in CFS patients. Additionally, the human herpesvirus 6 (HHV-6), a microbe which also causes CFS, can be integrated via *chromosomes*.[9] This virus can be active or inactive in a person's body.[10] This means that there's a possibility that the virus is inherited by a CFS patient but doesn't cause any harm to the health system. Thus, a patient should try to figure out whether he inherited CFS. Identifying the genetic potential of CFS enlightens experts as to why the patient has CFS in the first place.

Preexisting Immune Abnormalities

Chronic fatigue syndrome has a number of other medical names because of its oodles of unjustifiable causes. That being said, CFS is also known as chronic fatigue immune dysfunction syndrome because medical personnel also believe that the immune system could be a pivotal player in the explanation of the disorder. Some medical studies have discovered some preexisting (but not necessarily genetic) irregularities in the immune systems of patients diagnosed with CFS.[11]

Patients' immune systems respond inconsistently, sometimes over-reacting and other times underreacting. However, just like the other medical theories, this claim doesn't have any significant pattern that could justify the immune system idiosyncrasies as the actual roots of CFS. Medical research has also discovered that the majority of CFS patients have allergies to pollen, certain kinds of food, metals, and other types of substances. Just as is the case with the viral infection theory, allergies are a weak stand to explain the causes of CFS. Not all CFS patients are allergic, and neither do they all completely detest a distinct substance to which they're continually allergic.[12]

Psychiatric Causes

Other medical investigations affirm that chronic fatigue syndrome isn't a viral infection at all. It is said to be a psychiatric condition instead.[13] Extreme tiredness and inactivity are unexceptional symptoms found in CFS patients as well as in people suffering from some mental disability. At least half of CFS patients experience depression. This has led researchers to tie CFS to mental disorder.

Since some theories state that CFS is caused by genes that manage the body's response to traumatic events and injuries, medical researchers have also pondered that genes are unrelated to the conundrums of chronic fatigue. Instead, CFS could be just a condition of the patient's mind. This theory has been controversial for academic dons involved in CFS research. Many are displeased about labeling CFS as a "mental" illness, primarily because declaring CFS as a mental disorder dismisses the reality of CFS as a "real" disease for some. Still, the syndrome hasn't been proven to be a purely psychological sickness.[14]

Central Nervous System and Hormone Abnormalities

Research also indicates that the hypothalamus-pituitary-adrenal (HPA) axis could be a major factor causing CFS.[15] Hypothalamus-pituitary-adrenal disorder occurs when several chemicals in the brain system are at abnormal levels. This is significant for the study of CFS because the

HPA axis is responsible for several physical and emotional functions such as sleep, depression, and response to stress. All of these functions are related to the symptoms shown in chronic fatigue syndrome. A few of the more notable observations regarding this study are as follows:

- Significant changes in important neurotransmitters: CFS patients have been observed to have abnormally high levels of serotonin, a deficiency of dopamine, and an imbalance between the neurotransmitters norepinephrine and dopamine.
- Interrupted circadian rhythm: Almost all CFS patients have trouble with sleep, particularly in sleeping and waking. The circadian clock regulates the sleep-wake cycle and an exposure to viral infections can cause stress and trauma, disrupting this cycle. This leads to difficulty in getting much-needed rest.
- Deficiency of stress hormones: CFS patients have a low level of cortisol; this may explain why patients have a low tolerance to both physical and psychological stresses, such as a viral infection or even exercise.

Some CFS patients tend to look for a quick fix to resolve their hormonal tribulations. This means turning to over-the-counter (OTC) drugs and other quick remedies instead of making the change holistically, a change to all aspects of life, from social activities, diet, daily regimen, and finally, the cessation of bad habits. Weight gain and increased cortisol have been found to have a deeper connection with the level of stress that the CFS patient experiences. Cortisol has a significant role in the different bodily and metabolic processes affecting internal organs.[16]

Stress hormones, a category that includes adrenaline, provide one with instant energy along with other hormones such as cortisol and CRH. Otherwise known as corticotrophin releasing hormone, CRH is secreted from glands whenever a person faces a certain stressor or stressful event. This is in connection with the "fight or flight" mechanism that the CFS patient has when facing high levels of stress. An advanced level of adrenaline and CRH would then decrease the person's appetite; however, this would be only ephemeral. Cortisol would then help to replenish the lost minerals from the CFS sufferer's body after the stressful incident.[17]

Generally speaking, cortisol is the body's fight-or-flight hormone that's released every time one is stressed or faced with a certain stressor. Its main purpose is to replenish the lost energy after exertion during the fight-or-flight stage. It's the hormone responsible for letting the body revert back into its normal functioning after a stressful event. Ancestors of the human race, who could be traced to primitive man, needed this hormone to fight off wild beasts and to compete for food, shelter, and other basic necessities. At present, humans (whether CFS patients or not) still respond to stress by either facing it (the "fight" mechanism), or running away from the perceived threat.[18]

Stressors for the modern man are more complicated than those for the primitive bloke, and sometimes continual strain has a detrimental effect on the person's health. When cortisol is forfeited by glands, the body's viscera and tissues are relieved of stress, but continuous discharge of cortisol in this manner can be harmful. This is because cortisol is continually being discharged within the body in high amounts, which then predisposes the patient to develop other illnesses or conditions such as high blood pressure and diabetes mellitus, thereby compromising the body's verve to fight off infection.[19]

Low Blood Pressure

Another medical theory about the cause of CFS is the irregular blood pressure levels of patients. People who've been diagnosed with CFS also illustrate symptoms of neutrally mediated hypotension (NMH) that causes a dramatic drop in the patient's blood pressure level even during unpretentious motions such as standing up or moseying. This causes the patient to experience nausea, light-headedness, and proneness to fainting.[20]

RISK FACTORS

Similar to the medical theories explaining the causes of CFS, the risk factors are also quite vague. Listed risk factors encompass a very broad and general audience, making it seemingly possible for everyone to have CFS. Of course, not all individuals with the same symptoms may be diagnosed with the syndrome. As long as medical investigations regarding CFS are still active, there's no single risk factor that could guarantee the syndrome in an individual. The CDC says that more than one million people in the United States are diagnosed with chronic fatigue syndrome. This number is quite alarming considering that the complete lineup of risk factors is still unknown.[21]

Age, Gender, and Ethnicity

Chronic fatigue syndrome occurs in both sexes from all racial and ethnic groups. However, it's been observed that most of these CFS patients are between forty and fifty years old.[22] Studies also show that there are more women who suffer from CFS than men, even though the severity of pain doesn't differ from that of the men. Children and young adults may also have CFS but it isn't common. There are more girls diagnosed with the syndrome than boys.[23]

Psychological Risk Factors

Many chronic fatigue syndrome patients are ill with depression. It's one of the most common symptoms pooled among CFS sufferers. Social factors such as the individual's personality and mental health are said to influence the onset of CFS. Those who aren't able to tolerate stress and have experiences with depression have a higher chance of developing the syndrome.[24]

Although the medical disorders flanked by physical factors and emotional factors are still quite complex, scientific researchers have discovered that personality disorders are consistent among patients. This is momentous information. Compared to other indicators, depression seems to be the highest similarity among chronic fatigue patients. This could be a key lead for those investigating the risk factors of chronic fatigue syndrome.[25]

Stress

Psychological disabilities are promulgations for developing CFS, and researchers have also discovered relevant information regarding the patients' tolerance to stress. One of the possible causes of CFS includes a gene that handles the body's response to psychological tension. Studies have shown that patients who've experienced severe trauma and stress—especially those who've gone through a lot of abuse—are regrettably more prone to CFS.[26]

ANALYSIS

The complex nature of CFS makes the medical investigation of its causes and risk factors a challenging study requiring further examination. These factors not only differ on a case-to-case basis for every patient, but they're also quite common and may not even be related to CFS in the long haul. Nonetheless, the CFS patient must understand that not all hope is lost.

4

PATHOLOGY OF CHRONIC FATIGUE SYNDROME

Although pathology, by definition, pertains to diagnostics from a medical standpoint, diagnosis can present a discrete problem when it comes to chronic fatigue syndrome (CFS), because symptoms of the syndrome are similar to other medical complaints. There aren't any direct examination results that can verify the diagnosis, so confirmation of CFS involves a process of elimination.

GENERAL PATHOLOGY OF CFS

Chronic fatigue syndrome, as the name suggests, is characterized by persistent fatigue or exhaustion. Fatigue is the main indicator for this disorder, but not the type of fatigue a person faces after a gruesomely tiring or stressful day. It's not the type of tiredness that persists for only days, weeks, or couple of months.[1]

It's an intense, lingering, debilitating fatigue that can't be treated by a surefire set of medications, and it doesn't resolve through rest. It often becomes worse when a person does any kind of physical or mental activity. Pathologically, CFS totally affects a person's stamina and activity level. It results in a considerable lessening of an individual's work, school, personal, and social activities.[2]

Specific Set of Symptoms

An individual is said to be afflicted with CFS if he presents with three main symptoms. First, he has severe, extended fatigue for six or more successive months. Second, the fatigue notably affects the patient's daily physical work and routine. Third, the individual suffers four or more symptoms from a general list of symptoms of CFS.[3]

The first criterion is an extreme and continued fatigue that occurs for six months or longer and for 50 percent of the time.[4] There are also other guidelines released by the National Institute for Health and Care Excellence (NICE) stating that physicians should consider a diagnosis of CFS if a patient's fatigue level: (a) is relatively new to the patient or has a definite starting point, (b) is constant and or frequent, (c) cannot be explained by other conditions, (d) greatly affects the activities of a patient by diminishing strength to carry on daily activities both physical and mental, and (e) worsens after intense physical activity.[5]

The second criterion is where the individual experiences severe exhaustion while engaging in a typical activity. The individual may experience what's known as post-exertional malaise, or a period of extreme lethargy, and other CFS symptoms that persists for more than twenty-four hours. There's been ongoing research into this. Upon post-exertional malaise, there's a marked change in the blood and genetic manifestation.[6] This can be considered a basis for identifying CFS. The third criterion is that the individual experiences at least four of the identified general symptoms of CFS. These universal symptoms of CFS are:

- Neurocognitive issues, which may include short-term memory loss, clumsiness, difficulty in concentration and thinking, trouble in finding words or speech impairment, struggling with planning or organizing thoughts, and problems in processing information;
- Non-refreshing sleep or difficulty in sleeping, such as disrupted sleep, an unstable sleep-wake pattern, insomnia or hypersomnia;
- Muscle or joint pains without swelling or inflammation;
- Headaches differing in intensity, severity, or pattern;
- Painful or tender axillary or cervical lymph nodes; and
- Frequent sore throat.

Although the draining symptom of CFS is indeed fatigue, individuals often state that the mental deficiencies—including difficulty in concentration and memory loss—are the most upsetting. Some physicians posit that idled mental performance is due to depression, which is common in individuals with CFS. Aside from these symptoms, other general symptoms of CFS include the following:[7]

- Mental fogginess or a state of a clouded consciousness, wherein an abnormality is observed in the control of the level of consciousness that's milder than delirium;
- Sudden plunging blood pressure resulting in dizziness or nausea, paleness, fainting, difficulty in maintaining an upright position, and balance problems;
- Aggravating allergies including sensitivity to foods, noise, odor, light, medications, or chemicals;
- Irritable bowel syndrome including abdominal pain, stomachaches, bloating, diarrhea, or constipation;
- Incessant night sweats and chills;
- Visual disturbances including eye pain, blurring or worsening vision, light sensitivity, and dry eyes;
- Mental snags that may include mood swings, irritability, depression, panic attacks, and anxiety;
- Palpitations or escalated heart rate or shortness of breath (dyspnea);
- Chronic or a long-lasting cough;
- Recurring flulike illnesses that may or may not implicate chest pain; and
- Undetermined reasons for weight change (usually rapid weight loss).

Other Signs of Chronic Fatigue Syndrome

Apart from the symptoms of CFS listed above, there are specific biological signals found in most individuals with CFS. Notable changes affect the individual's central nervous system, hormones, and immune system. Many studies have connected chronic fatigue syndrome to the central nervous system. The nervous system is responsible for some important bodily functions such as slumber, response to stress, and depression. People with CFS have unusual levels of chemicals in the hypothalamus-pituitary-adrenal (HPA) axis, as elaborated in the preceding chapter.[8]

The hypothalamus decreases the production of corticotrophin discharging hormone, or cortisol, which is a steroid hormone released in reaction to stress, resulting in a reduction in the release of the pituitary gland, which then leads to *hypocortisolism*, or adrenal insufficiency. Mild hypocortisolism is one symptom consistently found in individuals with CFS, which may also explain the symptoms of slackened or weaker reaction to physical or psychological stresses, for instance, isometrics or infections.[9]

Neurotransmitters are chemical envoys of the brain. Other CFS signs noted are the changes in the major neurotransmitters, whereby patients have (a) remarkably high levels of serotonin, a compound supplying the sense of happiness and well-being, (b) deficits of dopamine, a neurotransmitter contributing to the sense of reward, or (c) inconsistencies between norepinephrine, a neurotransmitter responsible for attentive concentration, and dopamine. Studies also show that some individuals with CFS frequently exhibit disturbances in their sleep-wake cycles. The sleep-wake cycle is disciplined by the body's circadian clock, which is really a cluster of nerves found in the HPA axis. Stressful physical or mental events, such as illnesses or viral disease, can upset one's natural circadian rhythm. The inability to retune the circadian rhythm results in continual sleep instabilities.[10]

Some studies indicate that SPECT scans of individuals with CFS have diminished cerebral blood flow; PET scans have shown abridged metabolism of the brain; MRI scans have revealed the occurrence of small lesions.[11] These irregularities have been seen in clinical statuses of otherwise healthy folks. Anomalies in individuals with CFS most resemble those observed in AIDS encephalopathy.[12]

In addition, CFS is usually followed by substantial economic, social, and physical disability and dysfunction. Patients with CFS normally function at crucially lower levels, resulting in significant economic and personal stress. The high unemployment rates among the patients and the costs related to uninformed care are economic burdens faced by the patients that can result in depression. Chronic fatigue syndrome has been declared a form of infrequent depressive illness due to symptomatic overlaps.[13]

Signs of CFS in the Immune System

Scientific inquiries have shown that the immune system shows many abnormalities in individuals with chronic fatigue syndrome.[14] Some elements appear to be under-reactive, whereas others tend to be overreactive. Studies continue to spitball the theory that the majority of individuals with CFS have allergies to pollen, food, metal, chemicals, and other substances. One hypothesis posits that allergens, similar to viral diseases, may activate a series of immune system irregularities that are linked to CFS. However, not all people with allergies suffer from CFS. The risk outline for CFS is identical to the risk outline for some autoimmune diseases. These findings are mutable in that autoantibodies (antibodies that infect the body's own tissues) are present in those with CFS. Scientists found that the range of immunological deficiencies imply that CFS is a form of acquired immunodeficiency.[15]

Inconspicuous symptoms of chronic fatigue syndrome that may be logged from laboratory reports may include immunoglobulin G, immune complexes, alkaline phosphatase, low-level antinuclear antibody titer, cholesterol, lactate dehydrogenase, and atypical lymphocyte (a genus of white blood cell) levels.[16] There may also be a special type of fat manifest in CFS patients. These chronic phase lipids (CPLs) may be akin to "acute phase proteins" such as C-reactive protein, which escalates in settings of trauma and inflammation.[17]

Level of Symptoms

There are three levels of severity of chronic fatigue syndrome. First is a trifling presentation of symptoms, wherein an individual can take care of himself and perform light household tasks but with some difficulty. The patient might still report to work or go to school, but may often be absent periodically. It's likely that he's halted most social and leisurely outings, too. Days off from work or school and weekends are often spent reclining to recover from fatigue.[18]

Second is the moderate presentation of symptoms, wherein the individual experiences lessened agility and has limited ability in performing daily, routine tasks. The individual has difficulty sleeping at night and may experience other symptoms recurrently. Third is the severe presentation of symptoms, wherein the person can perform only nominal tasks daily. Any activity easily weathers the individual, and the symptoms experienced are heightened. He contends with mental processes such as concentrating. The CFS patient may require a wheelchair and won't be able to leave home most of the time. He might suffer from severe post-exertional malaise and may also be bedridden for long periods of time. He also becomes sensitive to noise, bright lights, odor, sounds, or what they call "overload phenomenon." The flexible cognitive, sensory, motor, or emotional overstrain may trigger a "crash," wherein the individual suffers an intense, debilitating mental and physical fatigue or weakness.[19]

Symptoms of Chronic Fatigue Syndrome in Men

In earlier epochs dating back to the 1800s, neurasthenia (currently referred to as CFS) consistently plagued men in upper class society. This was attributed to their hard work and society's overwhelming pressure combined with minimal time for sleep and rest. During this period, chronic fatigue syndrome was considered a male disorder.[20] However, over the course of time, more women were diagnosed with CFS than men.[21]

The common symptoms experienced by men are similar to those suffered by women, but skeptics believe men are hesitant to admit to symptoms such as muscle and joint pains, headache, malaise, and others. The reason for this is that men have more difficulty verbalizing their symptoms, probably due to gender stereotypes, their cultural and social upbringing, or their belief that the symptoms will just go away by themselves. Physicians are encouraging men to be more open in expressing their symptoms for prompter intervention.[22]

Symptoms of Chronic Fatigue Syndrome in Women

Symptomatically, there isn't much difference between chronic fatigue syndrome in women and men. Most women in their forties or fifties commonly mistake symptoms of menopause for CFS.[23] Some women with CFS report symptoms analogous to premenstrual syndrome. These include *dysmenorrhea*, pain felt in the lower abdomen, tension, irritability, headache, mood swings (emotional labiality), *dysphoria*, anxiety, stress, insomnia, tenderness in the breasts, bloating, constipation, and joint and muscle pain. It is possible that there are more women diagnosed with CFS than men because women are more likely to report symptoms of CFS early.[24]

Symptoms of Chronic Fatigue Syndrome in Children and Adolescents

A small percentage of children or adolescents are afflicted with chronic fatigue syndrome, since the age bracket during which CFS commonly occurs is usually between twenty and fifty years of age. Diagnosis of CFS in childhood happens rarely because children and adolescents seldom experience stress and anxiety, but it does happen, especially if the parents have a history of CFS themselves.[25]

CFS in children is usually detected between the ages of twelve and seventeen. Kids, like men, have a hard time voicing their symptoms due to difficulty in describing the nature or level of their fatigue or pain. Confirming a CFS diagnosis in children is different from that of adults, in that children must experience consistent occurrences of fatigue and the symptoms should last about three months (unlike adults, who must experience it for six consecutive months), and a pediatrician should be consulted at once.[26]

It is also more difficult to determine CFS in adolescents and children because they don't necessarily look ill, so it's sagacious to note the symptoms that they complain about. For most children and adolescents, the typical symptoms are headache, sleep troubles, and neurocognitive impairment. The headaches or migraine they experience are generally draining and accompanied by vomiting, shaking, diarrhea, abrupt declivity of body temperature, and severe debility.[27]

The neurocognitive deficiencies usually include difficulty in reading and focusing; some even have dyslexia that materializes only when the child is exhausted; and cognitive deficiencies worsen with any physical or mental activity. The variation and severity of symptoms tend to vary more swiftly and dramatically in children or adolescents than in adults. Many youngsters also show signs of juvenile fibromyalgia, or pain and sore points in nerve fibers and muscles. There are also some findings that show children or teenagers with CFS tend to have hyper-flexible joints.[28]

Other signs of note in a child with CFS are anxiety or refusal to go to school. It may also be difficult to differentiate CFS from other conditions in children such as infectious mononucleosis, psychiatric disorders, Lyme disease, and so forth. Chronic fatigue syndrome is often mistakenly branded as "school avoidance behavior" in children or as Munchausen's syndrome by substitution (a condition wherein a parent invents their child's sickness).[29]

RARE PATHOLOGY OF CHRONIC FATIGUE SYNDROME

There's a predetermined set of symptoms included in the evaluation for chronic fatigue syndrome and associated clinical perplexities. However, there are some individuals who demonstrate unusual pathology of the disease. Although these symptoms may be recognized, they're usually not omnipresent in CFS.

Brain Fog

Although brain fog or mental fog is a common symptom in individuals with CFS, its levels and severity vary. Other patients may feel the following:[30]

- Difficulty in word recall and use, which includes forgetting known words;
- Delayed recollection of names;
- Directional disorientation or inability to recognize familiar surroundings;
- Failure to recall where things are, as well as getting lost easily;
- Multitasking problems, which include failure to pay attention to more than one thing;
- Failure to remember the task at hand when sidetracked;
- Number problems, where the CFS patients experience difficulty in doing simple math, recalling sequences, and transposing digits.

Heart Abnormalities

Chronic fatigue syndrome, apart from being connected to nervous system, immune system, and hormonal dysfunctions, is conjoined with heart abnormalities as well. The following heart dysfunctions signal an onset of CFS: small left ventricle, low nocturnal heart rate inconsistency, quick QT interval, postural tachycardia, low blood volume, waning cardiac function, and irregular cardiac wall contraction. There are four chambers of the heart: the left ventricle, the right ventricle, the left atrium, and the right atrium. One study links an undersized left ventricle in a subgroup of CFS patients with a symptom known as orthostatic intolerance (OI).[31] According to this study, the individuals with OI have an undersized left ventricle that doesn't pump blood as steadily as it should, and this peculiarity is very distinguishable. Individuals who have OI usually feel dizzy while standing upright.

Blood pressure surges momentarily to oppose gravity and sustain the blood streaming to the brain when a person gets up from a lying or sitting position, but people with OI experience a drop in blood pressure when standing. This causes them to feel lightheaded, which at times can lead to semi-unconsciousness. Research has shown that an undersized small ventricle may increase the occurrence of OI and CFS symptoms due to the low blood flow to both body and brain. OI also was shown to be a precise subgroup of CFS.[32]

The sleep-wake configuration of people with CFS and their heart rates were observed overnight.[33] It was noted that low heart rate variability (HRV) was present in the individuals with CFS compared to a healthy group. When study members breathed in and out slowly, it was noted that the heart rate dithered, accelerating when breathing in and decelerating when breathing out.[34]

This is known as heart rate variability. Low HRV can denote (a) problems with the brain and nerve signals traveling to and from the heart, or (b) nuisances with the segment of the cardiac conduction system known as the sinus node. It was theorized that low HRV in CFS is related to the brain, since the autonomic nervous system controls the body's automatic functions. Deregulation of the autonomic nervous system is known as *dysautonomia* and is widely accepted among academics to be a characteristic of CFS.[35]

A common test concerning the heart's health is the EKG (electrocardiogram), wherein a machine plots the heart's electrical cycle on a graph. To be able to measure its specific characteristics, the points of the lines are marked. These intervals, or variances in points, provide useful information for doctors. The interval between points marked as Q and T is one of them. It was implied that a short QT interval rate, while uncommon in the general masses, is nearly ubiquitous in CFS patients because of its relevance to dysautonomia.[36] Another experiment also showed that QT intervals could differentiate cases of CFS from a similar disorder called fibromyalgia, with an 85 percent probability rate.[37]

Postural tachycardia is comparable to orthostatic intolerance, but it affects pulse rate rather than blood pressure. It's also linked to dysautonomia. Tachycardia is an unusually fast heart rate. Postural tachycardia therefore indicates that the heart rate increases irregularly upon standing. It is often observed as POTS, or postural orthostatic tachycardia syndrome, identified in individuals with CFS.[38] As a result of a research trial concerning the study of adolescents, CFS was deemed to be associated with symptomatic low vitamin D levels.[39] There are other speculative studies linking CFS to vitamin D deficiency.[40]

Investigators have noted that individuals with severe CFS have the lowest blood volume.[41] Further tests have shown that impaired heart function was a likely upshot of low blood volume and not due to structural deficiencies. Think tanks confer that low blood volume influences the many symptoms of CFS by removing oxygen from the cells, which they require to spawn energy, though this hasn't been confirmed by research.[42]

Furthermore, scientists have studied the correlation between irregular cardiac motion of the walls of the heart and CFS and examined the way the walls of the heart move to measure the success of treatment. However, the experts concentrated only on self-reported CFS subgroups. In the study, irregular motions (contract/relax) of the cardiac walls exist in some cases of CFS found with *cytomegalovirus* and Epstein-Barr virus infection.[43]

Other Rare Symptoms of Chronic Fatigue Syndrome

Other uncommon symptoms of CFS include the following:[44]

- Morning stiffness;
- Numbness;
- Earache;
- Prickly sensations in the hands or feet (paresthesia);
- *Temporomandibular joint (TMJ) disorder*;
- Sensitivity to the cold or heat that worsens the other symptoms;
- Recurring respiratory illnesses;
- Low fever or low temperature of the body;
- Too much sweating, dry mouth or eyes (sicca syndrome);
- Difficulty in moving the tongue;
- Disordered feelings of the tongue;
- Mouth ulceration;
- Painful or repeated urination;
- Rashes on the body;
- Tinnitus or humming, ringing, hissing, or popping noises heard inside both ears;
- Muscle spasms;
- Seizure;
- Canker sores;
- Persistent infections;
- Herpes or shingles.

Chronic fatigue syndrome can be a perplexing disorder and its pathology can be very difficult to ascertain. There are several tests to take, multiple benchmarks to meet, and several other sicknesses to rule out before anyone can be fully confirmed to be suffering from chronic fatigue. Symptoms should be carefully evaluated because CFS tends to coexist with other underlying illnesses. Although the main symptomatic feature of CFS is austere and incapacitating fatigue lasting for at least six months, the presence of other clues should be monitored as well to avoid mistaking CFS with other afflictions.[45]

It's important for patients and caregivers to note that additional research indicates that (a) orthostatic intolerance, which in some cases involves a virally-induced dysfunction of a patient's autonomic nervous system, (b) low red blood cell count and low plasma volume, (c) signs of left ventricular failure upon stress, and (d) left chamber damage when the patient is in an upright position, are among the prominent features and distinguishing patterns of CFS. Muscle weakness or delayed recovery of the muscles following exercise, orthostatic fainting, and de-creased cardiac output are just the tip of the iceberg when it comes to symptoms of chronic fatigue syndrome.[46]

ANALYSIS

In studying the pathology of CFS, it's vital to note the signs and symp-toms rather than to concentrate on the diagnosis. There's no standard laboratory test or *biomarker* for identifying CFS, thus the signs and symptoms present in an individual become the benchmarks for the diagnostic formulas delineated in the next chapter.

5

DIAGNOSING CHRONIC FATIGUE SYNDROME

Even though the fatigue isn't acute anymore, the chronic fatigue syndrome (CFS) patient is driven to change his lifestyle due to possible risk of relapse. Its incidence has taken its roots from both gene-to-gene relationships and environmental experiences. Various methods were used to decipher the spot-on root cause of CFS long ago, but these attempts were likely a failure. Most study designs are watered down with many possibilities, thus giving unreliable measures. With all the above in view, different attempts have been made to remove the obstacles and offer sound inferences and unified criteria for CFS diagnosis.[1]

Oxford University's criteria for chronic fatigue syndrome is similar to the diagnostic rules of the Centers for Disease Control and Prevention, except Oxford contends that the following should be excluded from diagnosis of CFS: patients with recognized medical situations with similar symptoms as those seen in CFS and in patients suffering from manic-depressive conditions, schizophrenia, eating disorders, longtime substance abuse, or other proven brain diseases.[2]

DIAGNOSIS AT A GLANCE

There aren't any specific diagnostic run-throughs for determining whether an individual has CFS, but there's an extensive process to be followed. First, the physician needs to acquire a detailed medical history of the patient through a string of questions. The CFS patient has to undergo a complete physical exam. Next, the patient has to pass a mental status examination through an interview.[3]

There are tests that assess the effects of fatigue on cognitive skills, such as mental organization, memory, and concentration. These evaluations can also be beneficial in differential diagnostic processes or for verifying specific areas where therapy would be gainful. Afterward, the patient is subjected to a standard series of laboratory tests, including blood and urine tests. Additional scans and tests might be required to dismiss other possible medical conditions. These may include the following:[4]

- Full blood count;
- Blood urea nitrogen (BUN);
- Blood biochemistry (calcium, sodium, potassium, urea);
- Creatine kinase (to exclude muscle disease);
- Blood glucose;
- Urinalysis;
- Alanine aminotransferase (ALT);
- Electrolytes;
- Globulin;
- Phosphorus;
- Total protein;
- Albumin;
- Alkaline phosphatase (ALP);
- Erythrocyte sedimentation rate (ESR);
- Thyroid stimulating hormone (TSH); and
- Transferrin saturation and other liver function tests.

Second-line tests may also be required, depending on the discretion of the physician, in case other illnesses are present as well. These include antibody diagnostic tests for certain disorders such as the following:[5]

- Hepatitis B or C;
- Lyme disease or Lyme borreliosis and parvovirus;
- Screening for celiac disease for inexplicable anemia;
- Gastrointestinal indications or evidence of malabsorption;
- MRI scan if additional neurological illnesses such as multiple sclerosis are noted on the basis of symptoms and signs;

- Autoimmune and rheumatology screens if joint and muscular pains are pronounced; and
- Pituitary and adrenal function tests if there are indications that imply a specific endocrine disorder.

Oftentimes, CFS diagnosis is a thorny mission for a number of reasons:

- The beginning may be gradual, after an individual has experienced an illness or stressful episode, or all of a sudden;
- The scope of the exposing symptoms is wide, and fatigue and pain may not always be notable;
- The individual may have been checked thoroughly but with negative findings for varying physical symptoms; and
- Complaints vary in category and intensity over a period of time (either weeks or months), which might confuse both the caregiver and the client.

Therefore, much of the diagnosis of CFS relies on the signs and symptoms presented by a patient.

Importance of Early Detection

Diagnosis of CFS is complicated because there aren't any sole lab tests, obvious indications, or inimitable biomarkers. Doctors must first rule out any other possible causes before diagnosing the patient with chronic fatigue syndrome. However, it's still important to detect CFS speedily if possible because it may lead to more severe psychological and physiological struggles.

Onset of CFS and Diagnosis

Careful scrutiny of the symptoms and the pattern of illness can establish a diagnosis of CFS. Simply put, CFS isn't something straightforward from a diagnostic standpoint like depression. It's a syndrome wherein fatigue is the foremost earmark affecting the mind and body. For a period of six months, the patient must be observed and for at least 50 percent of the time, he must be experiencing fatigue. Persons with clinical history of concurrent diseases are excluded from this diagnostic definition.[6]

Seventy-five percent of people suffering from CFS report acute viral infections such as bronchitis, gastroenteritis, tonsillitis, and meningitis.[7] Chronic fatigue syndrome may also arise from chicken pox, glandular fever, and rubella. It could also just be a derivative of vaccinations or toxin exposure. In the end, it isn't fair that patients are often left hanging by medical practice due to diagnostic uncertainty.[8]

If a patient experiences a viral infection, persistent fatigue that'll last for almost six weeks should be observed and considered for further diagnosis. If the symptoms persist four months, the patient should be diagnosed with CFS provisionally and an initial treatment approach can be made. After six months, the provisional diagnosis can be confirmed, and clinical procedures should be driven forward. Through this method, the onset of the illness can be monitored and an early working diagnosis can be established. With some cases, the onset of CFS can fail to kick off a warning. The disorder slowly eats the patient's well-being in an insidious manner, different from one that starts from an infection. The prescriber might not be able to initiate a test and the CFS patient himself may not be aware of deviations from his normal mental and physical state.[9]

A Patient's Experience

Treatment delays nurture frustration and severity of medical disorders. An unfit patient who registers a virus and hasn't received the right medical instruction will face a more classic range of symptoms and the physician may not be able to provide satisfactory explanation of the case. The absence of clear diagnostic supposition hinders the person from (a) the appropriate sickness benefits, (b) vital care, (c) precautionary measures, and (d) access and mobility of their needs. Around 25 percent of people with CFS are wheelchair bound, housebound, or even bedridden.[10]

A case study supporting the scrutiny of CFS as a "diagnosis of exclusion" occurred to a thirty-three-year-old man who for two years had been travailing with fatigue.[11] After two years of utilizing various modalities of clinical management, his suffering increased; later on, he was diagnosed with Lyme disease, which arose from a late infection associated with his CFS. He was unable to function well and became bed-bound. He didn't have a medical history of any disease and his health records were unremarkable. Late diagnosis of the disorder caused him to suffer drastic changes in his physical activities. The gentleman was a former police officer who practiced martial arts, yet his physical functionality deteriorated due to late detection. [12]

Reasons for Delayed Diagnosis

There are many reasons for late detection of CFS in a clinical setting. Most patients would think that their fatigue was bred by overwork, so they tend to rest for a period of time and then return to their former routine. In due course, they discover that they're ill, and their disorders might have grown severe as they neglected their well-being. The following notes elucidate delayed detection: [13]

- People might believe that CFS is a nonexistent disorder that isn't taught in medical school.
- Clinical specialists tend to dismiss the possibility of the disease and therefore don't recommend such a diagnosis.
- Clinical criteria for diagnosis aren't completely established. Published papers pertaining to CFS methods and treatment vary, and research designs are rigid for clinical practice.
- Lab tests aren't possible since there's no abnormality that can be spotted through any clinical procedure. The symptoms of CFS are neither unique nor specific.
- One major hindrance for early detection is that the symptoms should be observed for a minimum of six months until the physician can conclude the CFS patient's diagnosis.

THE PATIENT'S CLINICAL HISTORY

Assessment of the life events of the patient prior to the onset of CFS should be considered. The medical history of the CFS sufferer gives evidences for a more accurate medical diagnosis. In one experiment, nearly three hundred CFS patients said that they'd been sick for an average of sixty-three months before they were diagnosed with CFS. [14]

These people had been suffering with extreme stress that could have possibly contributed to their condition. Another study involved patients with infectious mononucleosis or upper respiratory tract infection initially, and, due to these adversities, development of chronic fatigue was made possible.[15] Additional health mishaps came from disorders of muscle function: *phonasthenia*, neurasthenia, and others concerning voice difficulties.[16] These studies occured during war, and the onset of the disease might have been triggered by trauma and psychological struggle.

Medical History of the CFS Sufferer

A patient's medical history may provide clues that lead to the development of chronic fatigue syndrome. The history also gives a clear picture of the nature and characteristics of the patient's symptoms. Moreover, the importance of the clinical history is related to subsequent steps advised by the doctor. The patient's history would also help to determine whether he's really experiencing CFS or if there's already a lingering condition exacerbated by CFS.[17]

For example, early stages of hepatitis might lead to CFS-like illness. Every ounce of blood taken out of the body and other tests performed are relevant key indicators for diagnosis. Lyme disease, which is often part of a CFS diagnosis, is induced by tick bites. Such a medical past can add to the complication of the diagnosis of CFS. Due to numerous factors (*psychosomatic*, etc.) and previous activities and uncertainty in the disease definition, CFS really needed a lot more studies before it finally became established in the medical community.[18]

Medical Overlaps in the Diagnostic Process

Chronic fatigue syndrome often occurs alongside fibromyalgia, a syndrome characterized by tender points throughout the body. Although the diagnostic characteristics of CFS and fibromyalgia are different, studies show that 20 to 70 percent of people with fibromyalgia have CFS.[19] Thus, researchers have considered that symptoms, patient characteristics, and treatments of functional somatic syndromes are manifestations of biomedical and psychosocial processes. The diagnostic overlays among these conditions can be explained by *pathophysiology*.

Therefore, the occurrence of one symptom might be able to expound the origins of another.[20]

Age and Early Life Factors in Diagnosis

Chronic fatigue syndrome doesn't choose the age of its victim. The syndrome can occur in adults and children alike. Pediatric settings may cause delay in diagnosing CFS among youngsters. Chronic fatigue syndrome at a young age is suggestive of early life causative factors, and the instigators of the disease might be difficult to identify, but their presence is definite from the beginning. These are considered environmental inducers.[21]

Early life inducers increase the potential of developing CFS during adulthood. Prenatal and neonatal exposure to the environment may induce some factors leading to development of CFS, as well. There are also studies fastening childhood autism with prenatal inflammatory attacks. Prenatal (before birth) exposure to disruptive chemicals associated with the *endocrine system* can induce aberrant responses of the immune system, thereby muddying the diagnostic steps of CFS even further.[22]

Role of the Immune System in Diagnosis

CFS detection and diagnosis needs a definite time frame in order to determine the "cause and effect" of the disorder. The likely causative factor of the onset of the disease might have occurred before the diagnosis of CFS. This leads to the fact that infectious agents, toxicants, viruses, or bacteria might already be present. This may mislead the medical findings and diagnostic results given to the patient. That in turn also evokes the assessment of blood levels of environmental chemicals and drugs and therefore pairs it with the postpartum biomarkers of CFS. Analyses suggest a strong correlation between the prenatal progress of the child and the critical window of the occurrence of CFS in later life.[23]

Heavy metals, lead, and polychlorinated biphenyls (PCB) are often found in the body during diagnosis. Clinical investigations concur that the toxicity induced by the chemicals causes an obtunded IQ. Lead is also demonstrable in blood. This lead-induced immune toxicity impedes some necessary body functions and can eventually lead to fatigue and other known CFS by-products. This is an important aspect to take into consideration diagnostically, since prenatal stages affect every dimension of childhood development.[24]

Immune dysfunction to date report facilitated abnormality across the *physiological* systems that have been appended by inflammatory cell damage during early life stages. It's also a result of stress, which is a postnatal stimuli of infections to which the CFS sufferer could have been exposed before.[25] Overall, immune dysfunction has an inordinate connection to CFS. Physiological systems can be interrupted by early life disruption of the *homeoregulatory* role of immunity cells in the neurons and endocrines.[26]

INTRODUCTION TO EXAMS, DIAGNOSTIC TESTS, AND SCREENING PROCEDURES

Prior to any diagnosis, examinations and diagnostic tests should always be performed. These tests are influenced by the medical history and other therapeutic procedures prescribed for the patient in the past.

Clinical Presentation

It's well founded that CFS is connected to recurring fatigue, but certain forms of fatigue (a) take shape after pre-illness conditions and (b) abruptly transpire a loss of energy to perform daily routines. Grown-ups with chronic fatigue syndrome have often experienced chronic headaches, difficulty in concentrating and other cognitive problems, attention deficit hyperactivity disorder (ADHD), interstitial cystitis, irritable bowel syndrome, sleep problems, and *temporomandibular joint (TMJ) disorder.*[27] Examinations or clinical procedures given to children are more likely based on the physiological attributes in growth such as any disruption in height, weight problems, disproportional size of the head, glandular or *tonsiliar enlargement*, evidence of chronic sinusitis, and *postural orthostatic tachycardia syndrome (POTS).*[28]

Clinical Evaluation

Although there isn't a single test that will provide a definitive CFS diagnosis, there are a lot of clinical evaluations recommended to eliminate other potential conditions, thereby marking CFS as the prime possibility. These methods are discussed later in this chapter, since these laboratory techniques often render unremarkable results.[29]

Diagnostic Tests and Screening Procedures

The following diagnostic tests are performed before a full CFS diagnosis is afforded by the physician.[30]

- Full blood count and differential;
- ESR or acute phase protein changes;
- Blood biochemistry;
- Creatinine kinase;
- Thyroid function tests;
- Liver function tests; and
- Urine tests for renal disease and diabetes.

Anything significant found in these tests will impact the patient's diagnosis and his syndrome will be reassessed. The second clutch of diagnostic tests must be performed. These procedures include:

- Antibody screening tests for infection such as hepatitis B and C, Lyme disease, and the presence of parvovirus should be checked. Positive results for any of these possibilities require immediate treatment.
- If gastrointestinal symptoms are prevalent, the patient must be screened for celiac disease. This may also be present if the patient is suffering from malabsorption and arcane *anemia*.
- Prominent joint pains might be present for patients who are elderly or older than forty. They can be screened using accurate rheumatology procedures.
- Neurological illness needs to be tested using an MRI scan to screen for signs of multiple sclerosis.
- Endocrine-related disorder should be verified through pituitary and adrenal function tests.

GENETIC TESTS

An important way to determine the cause, development, and progress of a medical condition is to know the genetic connection and environmental influences. Sundry studies have been made to demonstrate the connection between DNA and familiality with CFS. One study was based on the prevalence of the disease among family members.[31] Those with relatives suffering from CFS would likely have a higher risk of acquiring the same disorder. The subjects included twins ages fifty and older hailing from the Australian Twin Registry. Researchers found that fatigue can be hereditary when it occurs for a minimum duration of four weeks.[32]

In another study of twins with evidence of CFS, their data was used to examine nexuses of genetic involvement and DNA to chronic fatigue. Sustained fatigue and CFS-like illnesses should be probed based on the genetic and familial affinity factors. However, this situation might not be applicable for broader populations. There are several elements that need to be considered, including the due-process measures of fatigue, classification of CFS on the basis of environmental, social, emotional, and cultural setting, family interviews, and sampling within the family of each patient. Susceptible individuals are more likely to be those with genetic relation to those affected by the disorder.[33]

CENTRAL NERVOUS SYSTEM DIAGNOSTICS OF CFS

The central nervous system might be a system of defect as suggested by numerous CFS-related symptoms such as fatigue, impaired concentration, impaired attention, and short-term memory loss, along with headaches. Several diagnostic procedures can assess the functionality of the central nervous system, like neuroimaging, cognitive testing, neuropeptide assays, and autonomic assessment.[34]

Neuroimaging

Magnetic resonance imaging (MRI) is a method of seeing the brain's activities. This is done together with single photon-emission computed tomography (SPECT). Individuals facing trauma have fewer subcortical abnormalities compared to subjects with CFS. However, there are also dossiers that show the same MRI results among healthy and depressed people and CFS patients.[35] Using SPECT, researchers have found that people suffering from CFS have lower levels of local cerebral blood flow in the brain, unlike the healthy subjects.[36] *Hypoperfusion* is more evident in CFS patients compared to depressed subjects. However, another survey confirmed that cerebral blood flow for twins with chronic fatigue syndrome corresponds to the same blood flow of twins who are healthy.[37] Scientists believe that CFS has obvious abnormalities in the central nervous system. Conversely, this claim lacks functional significance and therefore remains inexplicit in the frontiers of medical science. Findings and more results are still awaiting further clarification and investigation.

Neuroendocrine Tests

CFS patients were found to have evidence of hypothalamic-pituitary-adrenal (HPA) axis. There is also some occurrence of serotonin pathways, which make stress. Hypocortisolism also exists in some patients. Genetic mutation has also been found in a family with thirty-two members suffering from CFS. The mutation impacts the body's production of globulin, a protein that's detectable during diagnosis, which helps in the transport of cortisol in the blood.[38]

Serum prolactin levels produced in CFS patients are greater than in those who are depressed but healthy. Unlike other acknowledged symptoms of CFS, HPA abnormalities, hormonal stress responses, and serotonin neurotransmission offer more evidence and certainty, though the findings aren't yet conclusive.[39]

Neuropsychiatric Tests

Some experts might believe that CFS is a psychiatric disorder. That's why doctors are sometimes reluctant to diagnose CFS. Chronic fatigue syndrome is actually related to various psychological disorders like somatization disorder, hypochondriasis, major depression, and atypical depression.[40] Obvious conditions for CFS patients are mood swings, which can last for a lifetime. Clinical studies note that chronically ill

CFS patients have current and lifetime major depression.[41] There are also high rates of anxiety disorders preceding the onset of CFS.[42]

Management of the patients with respect to diagnostic tests is imperative even when it comes to CFS sufferers without psychiatric issues. This helps physicians rule out other symptoms and may also be a way to assess any issues of maladaptive coping styles, psychopathological situations, and psychiatric disorders. Soon, this could be an integral part of the clinical evaluation for every patient.

Furthermore, cognitive problems involving attention, concentration, and memory malfunction are some of the disruptive and unsettling traits of CFS. Patients suffer with discrepancies in processing information, poor learning, and memory loss. Thus, the patients would have a gritty time with cognitive information processing, leading to poor performance on the job or elsewhere. This leads to suspicions that CFS can be associated to psychological impairment or psychiatric disorder. Despite all this, there are also countless cases where CFS patients show highly intellectual abilities and normal cognitive performance during the diagnostic process.[43]

One way of checking the patients who are affected by CFS is by use of exercise programs and cognitive therapy. This is based on the possibility that behavior and cognition play a major part in CFS diagnosis. These are all based on ruminant association of the symptoms to the disease. Thus, cognitive therapies are also readied to test the patients. Chronic fatigue syndrome sufferers undergoing advanced behavior therapy have shown applicable results of stagnated pain in the lower back as well as in the chest, and they can perform better coping exercises.[44]

Sleep Tests

Sleeping pattern is a highly overlooked periphery of CFS diagnosis. Sleep is the unrivaled form of rest. People with fatigue are short of rest, and sleep can be one of the symptoms or drawbacks of being ill with the syndrome. Chronic fatigue syndrome patients have difficulty in their sleeping patterns, various sleeping disruptions, and inconsistent napping routines compared to healthy people. This is a highly observable piece of the diagnostic puzzle. Experts have found that CFS patients have *alpha-intrusion* that occurs during *non-REM sleep*. However, some studies didn't yield similar results. There are also cases where patients with CFS-like illness have been found to have a sleeping disorder called apnea, a condition that can be treated immediately, excluding any possibility of CFS.[45]

IMMUNOLOGICAL TESTS OF CFS

Compared to a healthy person, CFS sufferers have been observed as having superfluous quantities of *autoantibodies*. This results in a sapped immune system and low levels of protection against foreign "invaders." The magnitude of the physical degradation, cognitive deficiencies, and physiological impairment is due to the body's inability to fight these conditions. Thus, there's a great need to check the antibody count and to provide the CFS patient with the necessary antibodies that can fight his specific symptoms. Immunological tests to date aren't yet fully established in the clinical arena.[46]

Infectious Agent Screening

Although the Epstein-Barr virus has been indirectly connected to CFS, medical researchers have been trying to solidify a viral connection. However, there's still no tangible evidence to support the idea.[47] It's improbable for a CFS patient to have only one source of infection, so this arena must be scrutinized and scientists must delve more closely into it for immunological hints regarding the disorder.

ANALYSIS

Cast-iron certainty of diagnostic results still lies afar. Researchers and the medical world continue to investigate how to clarify and support the diagnosis of CFS. In fact, difficulty in the diagnosis of CFS could arise from inadequate and poorly described sampling procedures, and sometimes the choice of comparison groups simply isn't diverse enough to draw conclusions. In summary, the diagnosis for this illness is established on the foundation of subjective clinical interpretation, exclusion, and the CFS client's rapport with the caregiver.

6

ROLES OF THE FAMILY PHYSICIAN, INTERNIST, AND NEUROLOGIST IN CHRONIC FATIGUE SYNDROME

A physician is necessary to ensure the wellness of a patient with chronic fatigue syndrome (CFS). However, a doctor's role in regard to treating this syndrome must be clearly defined before seeking medical attention. This chapter is about the importance of finding the right physician and identifying the appropriate questions to ask. The research presented here discusses the usual functions of the three physicians who normally handle CFS cases—the family physician, the internist, and the neurologist—and also enumerates the questions a CFS patient should ask his healthcare professionals. Likewise, the following paragraphs also include possible questions a physician might ask a person who has CFS.[1]

COMMON FUNCTIONS

The basic task of any physician depends on the education he's completed. People with CFS should learn about the roles played by their various physicians prior to their consultations in order to prevent misunderstandings and incorrect assumptions. This section defines the roles of a family physician, an internist, and a neurologist.[2]

Family Medicine and CFS

A family physician is known to be a practitioner in general medicine. This doctor has wide medical training that can be of use to a diverse set of patients (including CFS sufferers) to provide primary care.[3] This means that a family physician has the ability to provide initial medical attention to anyone. Considered the backbone of the community health system, a family physician attends to any health concern that the CFS sufferer may have, whether it's a physical, mental, or emotional topic.[4]

Since a family doctor has knowledge about wide spectrum of medical areas, he's well-rounded in handling various maladies. Moreover, when it comes to CFS, one of the basic roles of a family physician is to prevent further illness of the patient.[5] An awareness about general medicine enables a family physician to guide patients to a proper and healthy lifestyle. As the family physician establishes a CFS patient's healthy immune system, he lessens the chances that the patient will suffer from other clinical disorders.

A family physician also acts as a role model who promotes professional attire, appropriate behavior, correct posture, proper speech, and auspicious habits in terms of health.[6] This helps the members of the community in attaining a healthy physical condition and well-being. Aside from assuring the patient's wellness, a family physician continually provides a personal patient-physician connection.[7] The profound relationship between a physician and a patient develops over the course of time, as a physician may treat his patient from birth to adulthood. This role enables the doctor to track and record the medical history of the CFS patient wholeheartedly.

Another function of a family physician is to refer and advocate specialists for his patients when necessary.[8] Depending on the complexity of the health concern of a patient, the family physician may seek the help of an appropriate specialist with across-the-board knowledge of a specific area of medicine. The family physician serves as a channel between two parties: the client and the specialist. Since a family doctor usually handles the primary record of the CFS client, this physician can provide important information that may help the specialist. At the same time, the family physician can help a patient to comprehend the specialist's findings by explaining them in simple terms.[9]

Internists and CFS

Contrary to a family physician's wide range of patients, an internist focuses only on adults. Thus, an internist is often referred to as a doctor for grown-ups.[10] The core of an internist's medical training is an expansive field called adult medicine.

An internist practices almost all the basic functions of a family physician because an internist is also knowledgeable in general medicine. The family physician's role, such as maintaining and improving the quality of a patient's health, are also performed by an internist.[11] Enhancing the well-being of a person encompasses the prevention, immediate discovery, and treatment of a health problem such as chronic fatigue syndrome in a mature adult patient. Nonetheless, an internist implements a more scientific and logical approach when diagnosing a specific health concern.[12]

Aside from his knowledge of general medicine, an internist also has subspecialties of his choice.[13] Possible subspecialties include neurology, immunology, cardiology, ophthalmology, gastroenterology, dermatology, and many others.[14] An internist's métier provides deeper knowledge into a specific medical field, which in turn enables him to handle the more complex health concerns of CFS patients.

Most of the time, an internist acts as a consultant to other doctors such as surgeons, the family physician, and other specialists. These doctors refer their patients to an internist who can analyze serious medical issues. Due to a vast and more in-depth background in medicine, the internist can expertly evaluate the clinical indicators reported by his adult CFS patient. In addition to handling referrals, internists also assess whether a patient qualifies for surgery.[15]

Internists may attend to patients who are planning to undergo a surgery at the request of a surgeon or a family physician.[16] This role requires explanation of the potential risk of the surgery, preparing the CFS patient prior to the operation, and assisting the client after the surgical process.[17] Based on a study, an internist usually tries to reduce the patient's surgical danger when there's about 65 percent or more risk of CFS perceived.[18] This corroborates that an adult patient should consult with an internist to diminish the possible threat of surgery.

Neurologists and CFS

Disorders involving the nervous system are commonly treated by a neurologist.[19] This physician has a medical expertise that focuses on diagnosing and managing the CFS patient's nerves, whether the problem involves the central or peripheral nervous system. In addition, a neurologist can have a diverse set of patients since this physician treats the neurological concerns of adults as well as children.[20]

Similar to a family physician and an internist, a neurologist is also conversant in general medicine.[21] This enables the neurologist to assess the health concerns of a CFS patient. However, a neurologist can provide a more thorough evaluation of the medical issues related to neurology. When a patient has a neurological issue such as Alzheimer's disease, peripheral nerve disorder, brain tumors, Parkinson's disease, or sleep disorders, a neurologist serves as the primary care provider for the patient.[22] As a primary care specialist, a neurologist has the overall control in managing the patient's health.

The neurologist also examines the cognitive ability of a patient.[23] This role involves testing the CFS sufferer's mathematical logic, memory, and language capacity to determine the condition of his motor system, cranial nerves, and sensory system.[24] Identifying the cognitive ability of a patient helps the neurologist to understand the patient's situation. In terms of diagnostic examinations, a neurologist also serves as a patient's guide.[25] This physician may request blood tests, electroencephalography, biopsy, spinal fluid analysis, and imaging tests.[26] The findings of the diagnostic examinations clarify the condition of the patient. With these diagnostic results, a neurologist gives a more comprehensive analysis of the patient's health situation. When a neurologist finally identifies the extent of the CFS patient's nerve-related disorder, he forms a plan on how to pursue treatment.[27] This protocol enables the patient to recover from his neurological issue. Depending on the patient's condition, the neurologist may include a recommendation for surgery.[28] This means that another role of a neurologist is to refer the CFS patient to a neurosurgeon as necessary.

QUESTIONS FOR THE DOCTOR

When a doctor diagnoses a patient with chronic fatigue syndrome, the patient should ask some questions to completely understand his health condition. Aside from knowing the definition of this syndrome, individuals with CFS must also learn about its causes and treatment from a physician. The following section outlines some of the potential questions a CFS patient may ask a family physician, an internist, or a neurologist, as well as explaining why such questions must be asked by a patient.

"What Causes CFS?"

According to a study of 1,000 participants, about 8.5 percent had unbearable fatigue for at least six months without any clear justification.[29] Thus, it's essential for the patient to ask the specific cause of his syndrome to identify why he's affected by CFS. Some of the common viruses presumed to initiate CFS are Epstein-Barr, varicella-zoster, hepatitis B, and *mycoplasma pneumoniae*.[30] A patient with CFS may ask his physician if any of these viruses caused his syndrome. Another question that can be raised to a physician is in regard to the potential ways of acquiring viruses that cause CFS. Aside from viruses, an uncharacteristic immune system and hormonal problems may also be factors related to chronic fatigue.[31] Discovering the possible reasons behind CFS is also important for a patient to prevent such disease in the future.

"Is CFS Inherited?"

Since a family physician usually tracks the medical history of a patient and his family record, this physician is the most appropriate doctor to ask this. A family doctor can access a CFS patient's medical archives to determine if the patient's CFS is hereditary. This question is also crucial in diagnosing the immediate family members of the patient. In this way, the syndrome can be immediately eliminated.[32]

"What Are the Symptoms and Consequences of Having CFS?"

The most common symptom of CFS is, of course, fatigue, which can't be cured with bed rest and continues for a minimum of six months.[33] Depending on the severity of the syndrome, the symptoms from one patient to another vary, yet another reason why the CFS patient should ask his doctor about them. Further consequences of CFS include headache, muscle pain, inability to concentrate, enlarged lymph nodes in the neck or armpit, sore throat, memory loss, difficulty in sleeping, and joint pain.[34] A CFS patient may also be angry, frustrated, and depressed.[35] If a CFS sufferer is made aware of these symptoms, he'll be prepared should they materialize.

"What Other Diseases Are Related to CFS?"

Chronic fatigue syndrome can also occur together with other illnesses.[36] Other than fatigue, a patient with CFS should also ask about illnesses related to the syndrome. This information is quintessential in preventing other health issues in a CFS patient. Based on a study, CFS might be related to blood-brain barrier permeability (BBBP).[37] A CFS patient may ask a neurologist if his syndrome has a connection to BBBP and if it can cause another neurological quagmire.

This enables the patient to manage or prevent other potential health concerns regarding his nervous system health. CFS is also associated with fibromyalgia and Gulf War syndrome, which are both related to long-term fatigue.[38] A CFS patient may also ask a physician if he has a risk of having those disorders. Another purpose of this question is for the physician to treat not only the syndrome, but also the patient's other health problems at the same time.[39]

"What Are the Possible Ways to Treat CFS?"

Some of the common treatments for CFS are cognitive behavior therapy, exercise programs, and pharmacological therapy.[40] A CFS patient must know which specific medical plan suits him. The patient may also ask a family physician, an internist, or a neurologist about the appropriate person to provide such treatment. It's always better to seek a physician's advice regarding the treatment instead of using alternative therapies, such as an exclusion diet and aromatherapy.[41] Such alternative therapies pose a higher risk and the potential for harm. Recommendations from healthcare professionals like family doctors, internists, and neurologists are more trustworthy and reliable.

A patient can also ask his healthcare provider about possible medications. Since a CFS patient often suffers from unbearable pain, he may ask for pain relievers for immediate and temporary relief. Based on the patient's treatment plan, a physician knows if temporary medication is necessary. If medicine is prohibited, a patient may solicit advice from the physician about other methods of reducing pain. Preparing a treatment plan may take days, thus it's important for a patient to have a reprieve when necessary. Exhausting all the suitable CFS treatments also gives the patients better alternatives to choose from. In addition, a patient can set his schedule in accordance to the medical treatment once a treatment regimen has been established.[42]

"How Is the Improvement of the CFS Patient Measured?"

There isn't any blood test or recognizable physical condition that determines the improvement of a CFS patient.[43] Thus, the patient should ask the physician for a tangible way to measure the progress of his treatment. Questionnaires, roundtables with the patient, and a patient's self-records are some of the tools that can be used to assess the CFS sufferer's response to medical treatment.[44] A CFS patient may also inquire about the frequency of conducting these assessments. Identifying the right tool and its occurrence enables the CFS patient to prepare for his recovery, and questions about health progress also help the patient to understand the goal of the medication schemata.

"Are Support Groups Necessary?"

Depending on the CFS patient's situation, a physician may recommend a support group, which is a valuable resource for all.[45] It's best to ask if this pack of friends is mandated for a specific patient. Just as symptoms vary from one patient to another, so does the sine qua non for a support group. For a child with CFS, a family physician who's also well-rounded in pediatrics can offer emotional support. According to a study, constant pediatric support lessens symptoms during the child's recovery period.[46]

"Is a CFS Patient Considered a Fully Disabled Person?"

In medico-legal terms, a CFS patient who is disabled for years and who shows less than 10 to 20 percent improvement over the course of ten years is considered to be permanently disabled.[47] In some cases, CFS isn't qualified as an unending disability when a patient shows progressive improvement.[48] A CFS patient should know if his condition can be considered as a disability. It's important for a patient to be aware of his eligibility for medical disability benefits. If necessary, a client may also ask the attending physician to issue the required clinical papers to validate the degree of injury.

QUESTIONS FOR THE PATIENT

A patient with CFS should also be prepared for the questions that a physician may ask. The following sections outline topics that may arise during the consultation with a family physician, an internist, or a neurologist. These are the questions necessary for an in-depth exploration of a patient's CFS. It's useful for the CFS sufferer to be aware of these inquiries prior to the appointment with the physician. Preparation leads to a more productive medical consultation for both the patient and doctor.[49]

"What Are the Symptoms Currently Experienced?"

Even if a client is already diagnosed with CFS, a physician may still ask this question to monitor the patient's condition. This question covers all of the patient's unusual and unbearable symptoms. Since CFS shares similar medical signs with other illnesses, a physician may ask the CFS patient to divulge such information to immediately eliminate other related diseases or to confirm a CFS diagnosis.[50]

"For How Long and How Often Are the Symptoms Experienced?"

Intolerable fatigue is considered "chronic" only when it lasts more than six months.[51] This means that tiredness over the course of a month or two may not be classified as chronic fatigue syndrome. It also proves that the duration of the symptom is crucial for evaluating the extent of CFS. Aside from identifying the nature of the symptoms experienced by the patient, the time period and frequency of the patient's CFS symptoms are also the physician's concern when analyzing the syndrome.[52]

A family physician or an internist also asks this question in order to monitor the development of a patient. By asking this question, the doctor expects the CFS patient to be able to identify how long or how frequently the symptoms occur. As a follow-up question, a physician may also ask when the patient experienced the symptom. This information determines not only the duration and frequency, but also the time of the day of the symptom's occurrence.[53]

"Does the Patient Also Have a Family Member with CFS?"

This question may arise during the initial consultation when attending doctor isn't the patient's regular family physician. Chronic fatigue syndrome can be genetically inherited by a person, so knowing the family's medical history enables the physician to confirm the probable cause of the syndrome. In addition, the doctor may also ask how the patient's relative recovered from CFS.[54]

He may opt to follow the same procedure adopted by the patient's relative who successfully recovered. If the treatment for the patient's relative doesn't work, the healthcare professional may amend the treatment that was proposed in the past. This question helps the physician formulate possible ways to manage the sufferer's condition. The inquiry is unnecessary when the attending physician is the family's longtime doctor, since that ensures the patient's medical history is known.[55]

"Was Trauma Experienced in the Past?"

Traumatic situations such as medical operations or severe accidents are identified to cause CFS.[56] A physician needs to ask this question to determine whether traumatic events led to a patient's syndrome. The physician presents this question not only to the patient, but also to the patient's family, since a patient may not remember or be aware of some traumatic events if they occurred long ago or while the patient was still a juvenile. In this situation, the physician's only resource is the patient's family members, specifically the parents who witnessed the growth of the patient.[57]

This question helps the physician to figure out the cause of the client's syndrome. Another purpose of the question is to record such traumatic events that may help in the recovery process. For an exhaustive analysis, the physician may also ask follow-up questions to learn more about his patient's health status. The doctor may study the patient's tragic experience and analyze how to minimize its effect on the life situation of the patient.[58]

"Does the Medical Treatment Suit the Patient's Schedule?"

The treatment plan is arranged and set by the doctor, but he generally asks this question to be considerate. If a physician organized a treatment schedule without consulting the patient, it is possible that the allotted time of the physician may not complement the patient's daily schedule. Identifying the availability of the patient assists the physician in constructing an attainable medical plan for the CFS sufferer.[59]

"Is Treatment Affordable for the Patient?"

The medical treatments for CFS are usually expensive.[60] This question ensures that the physician builds a treatment plan that's affordable for the CFS patient. Financial status should be considered prior to treatment planning. It's possible that the money prepared by the patient for his consultation is much less than the amount later realized. For improved fee arrangements, the physician might ask his patient to identify the specific amount of money dedicated for treating the CFS. This question also resolves the possible problem regarding money matters between the patient and the physician.[61]

ANALYSIS

When all is said and done, the roles of a family physician, an internist, and a neurologist are vital to an individual with CFS. These physicians have commonalities in terms of conventional functions but still make distinct contributions to the patient's medical development. There are cases where patients who have severe symptoms of CFS become so dependent on other people that they become housebound or bedbound. Access to healthcare services may be laden if the professionals involved such as internists, family physicians, and neurologists aren't well-informed about the possible attitudes of their patients toward them. Unfortunately, the skeptical attitudes of these caregivers may cause further suffering to CFS patients.

7

ROLE OF THE HOSPITAL IN CHRONIC FATIGUE SYNDROME

Due to its persistent recurrence of symptoms, chronic fatigue syndrome (CFS) requires delicate, continual, and appropriate treatment by the hospital. Besides the support received from the patient's family, hospitals with professional staff and the proper facilities also play a big role in the physical and psychological treatment of people who deal with this disorder. The hospital is often responsible for the diagnosis of the patient's condition.[1]

Chronic fatigue syndrome patients don't usually look as sick as they may feel. That's why friends, family members, and others may not always take a CFS patient's complaints seriously. During these times, *hospitalists*, who try to properly understand the patient's experience and provide an accurate diagnosis and the proper care required for their condition, can become a lifeline for the CFS patient. Hospitalists also provide a sense of hope for the CFS sufferer.[2]

HOSPITALS AND PATIENT-DOCTOR INTERACTION

Hospitals provide treatment such as cognitive behavioral therapy (CBT) and psychiatric consultations. This kind of medical treatment involves a series of one-hour sessions that focuses on discussing the nature of the patient's illness and the behaviors that may get in the way of the recovery.[3] Although CBT can only prevent the occurrence of some of the symptoms, studies have shown that the cognitive behavioral therapy performed in hospitals greatly influences a patient's improvement in terms of self-esteem and social interaction. Besides CBT, graded exercise therapy—a course of action often found in hospitals—and medications also contribute to diminishing the symptoms of CFS.[4]

Personal medical treatment aside, hospital care environments also contribute a great deal to the well-being of CFS sufferers along with other patients who experience different kinds of illnesses. A 2008 survey revealed the importance of a proper hospital environment for the betterment of its patients.[5] In their studies, researchers noted the effects of factors such as the number of educated staff and the quality of the hospital's facilities on the mortality rate and well-being of the patients residing on hospital grounds. Not surprisingly, data showed higher mortality rates in the hospitals with lesser staff and facilities.[6]

Research proves that better healthcare ambience enhances patient self-improvement, which is needed by CFS patients who are confused by their current state and troubled by the fact that the origin of the disease can't be precisely verified. This applies not only to CFS patients, but to others, too, such as cancer patients. Being in an environment where people share similar experiences helps CFS patients to understand how to deal with what they're experiencing and to realize that they're not alone.[7]

Hospitals and their staff—notwithstanding the medical services that they provide to their patients (like those who suffer from CFS)—also offer social interaction and reassurance to their clients. That's not always easy to do, as the patient is often in a threadbare state of mind in such a setting, but even the slightest encouragement can lead to positive changes.[8] At this point, the CFS patient learns to trust the hospital. If not, there won't be much progress. The healthcare professional at the hospital stands as a reflection of a friend who a patient can rely on and take advice from, thereby meaningfully boosting the patient's level of social interaction.[9]

In general, a hospital's contribution to its CFS patients and others includes not only the medical treatment for their disorders or diseases, but also a certain level of emotional and social support. The patient-doctor interface helps boost the sufferer's outlook on his condition. This psychological stimulation, delivered by various counseling and physical and psychological treatments, improves the patient's quality of life despite his disorder. Also, the hospital provides a secure environment where CFS clients can interact without being worried about their condition or about being criticized by others, as well as a complete facility to ensure the proper amount of determination required for an individual to improve both physically and mentally. [10]

CFS SETTINGS: INPATIENT VS. OUTPATIENT

In brief, an inpatient is someone who receives treatment requiring him to stay on hospital premises, whereas an outpatient obtains medical assistance beyond hospitals, whether at his home or in a doctor's office. Because there isn't a cure for CFS at present, both inpatient and outpatient methods are used to ease the symptoms caused by this disorder. [11]

In an inpatient setting, the CFS patient's medical condition is continually monitored and treated. Outpatient care, on the other hand, can integrate diverse forms of treatment such as family sessions, graded activities, and exercise programs that involve trainers or physiotherapists whose goal is to reestablish the client's self-esteem. Since CFS is to some degree both a physical and a psychological disorder (since factors such as stress are also involved), the inpatient setting relies more on the patient-doctor interaction represented by firsthand counseling by medical specialists. The outpatient setting ferries more of the approach outside of the hospital. [12]

Inpatient Setting

The severity of the patient's condition determines whether an inpatient setting is appropriate for a CFS patient. Most likely, people with moderate to very severe levels of fatigue will be subjected to intensive monitoring and care. The different clinical strata of fatigue are described in many works of research. [13]

Moderate fatigue is the level at which the patient has reduced mobility and is restricted from some activities in his daily life. Most likely, people with moderate fatigue would have to stop work and are required to have many rest periods. Patients with severe cases have the ability to carry out only the minimal tasks of daily living, such as washing their faces, and they rely on wheelchairs for mobility. In very severe cases, individuals are bedridden and immobilized due to fatigue. The hospital then would need to admit the patient, who would undergo unremitting monitoring.[14]

Inpatient settings are abundant in larger urban hospitals and fewer in smaller, rural hospitals.[15] A CFS patient in an inpatient setting commonly receives medication to help ease the effects of the symptoms. A comprehensive care package, such as one that includes treatment as well as follow-up rehabilitation, would be appropriate to describe this setting. In an event where the person can no longer perform daily tasks, the hospital rehabilitates him to regain strength and to recover by providing counseling and by prescribing treatments such as graded exercises accompanied by workout management strategies, sleep supervision, or relaxation techniques, as well as proper medications for relieving the pain caused by other conditions such as fibromyalgia.[16]

Among the various hospital treatments, stress and sleep management as well as psychological healing and exercise regimens are beneficial among CFS patients. In a hospital setting for CFS patients, it's first determined if stress management is applicable for the patient. This goes for the rest of the possible treatments considered. Chronic fatigue syndrome naturally manifests immobility and sudden fatigue, although in an inpatient setting, treatments promoting physical movements are often endorsed. The reason for this is that the significant decrease in muscular strength and agility results from the patient's moderate amount of physical activity.[17]

Outpatient Setting

Outpatient settings could also be termed *home health care*. In the past, home health care, or the outpatient setting, was a treatment normally associated with family members taking care of their ill, along with nurses assisting the family and providing for the proper medical care required by the patient, in their own homes. Delivering professional nursing services to patients' homes has now become more in demand, wider in range, and complex as manifested by the conditions of CFS. Some factors have greatly contributed to the changes in the home care trend:[18]

- Rising costs of medical care;

- A growing population of elderly people;
- A continually rising need to manage chronic disorders;
- Preventing illnesses; and
- Enhancing patients' quality of life.

In the past, home health care began when the client was discharged by the hospital. Nowadays, outpatient care has morphed into a way to avoid hospitalization.[19] Outpatient settings most likely involve the intervention of physical therapists for nonhospital activities as well as the family members. The hourly sessions provided by cognitive behavioral therapy also endure in this type of setting since the patient doesn't require admission to the hospital. He's given counseling to regain confidence that may have been affected by the lack of social involvement due to the symptoms of fatigue brought about by CFS.[20]

Family sessions also count as outpatient resolutions. With this approach, the patient is counseled along with his family. The CFS patient's current condition is explained to the whole family in order to introduce them to lifestyle changes he might require. The sessions are concerned with task management issues such as organizing schoolwork, reintegrating exercise into daily life, reestablishing the patient's normal sleeping routines, helping relatives with social issues, and assisting the family in restoring some sense of normalcy to their family life.[21]

Graded activities and exercise programs are also used in outpatient settings. These activities focus on bridging the gap between the patient's current physical condition and the physical ability required to accomplish the basic tasks of daily living. The kinds of programs initiated in these treatments are also decided by the patient and his family at the same time. Patients and caregivers should also take note of which setting (inpatient vs. outpatient) has a more positive effect on the patient's lifestyle, the kind of medical disorder he's experiencing, and primary factors affecting the occurrence of his symptoms.[22]

QUALITY OF HOSPITAL CARE VS. OUTCOME OF TREATMENT

The quality of hospital care hinges on health care delivery and how the staff manages the patients. Since CFS patients aren't the only population in the hospital warranting medical assistance, other clients must also be accounted for. The elderly, most especially, are high priorities in a hospital setting. It's estimated that by 2020 the number of U.S. adults over the age of sixty-five will be more than 53 million, with many of those being CFS sufferers.[23]

This means that there'll be a higher occurrence of other kinds of illnesses that a hospital must prioritize. Just as with CFS patients, older people require monitoring and psychological support because they too need to feel as if they're still a part of the community.[24] This affects the quality of health care that CFS patients are subjected to. Since their condition also requires continual monitoring, psychological assistance, and care as well as rehabilitation, a hospital must be able to provide appropriate services for all patients regardless of the medical condition in question.

Uneven distribution of amenities can also be a serious problem in terms of quality health care for individuals who have CFS. Two facets of this problem are (a) unequal distribution of care, and (b) increasing specialization. In some areas, particularly remote and rural locations, there are insufficient healthcare professionals and services available to meet the needs of individuals. Ruralized CFS clients may need to drive sizable distances for the services they require. Furthermore, an increasing number of healthcare personnel provide specialized services.[25]

Specialization can lead to fragmentation of care and often to increased cost, which can be a problem for CFS patients who aren't financially stable or capable, considering their disorder may have reduced greatly their economic support. To patients, this may mean receiving care from anywhere from five to thirty people during a hospital stay. This seemingly endless stream of personnel is often confusing and frightening and may greatly affect the hospital care of CFS sufferers.[26]

Another problem concerning the quality of health care that CFS patients receive is access to health care itself. This concerns not being able to have health insurance. Absence of health insurance is connected to low income, which has a great effect on CFS sufferers incapable of sufficient mobility. Low income has been associated with (a) relatively higher rates of infectious diseases such as tuberculosis and AIDS, (b) problems such as substance abuse, rape, and violence, and (c) chronic diseases or disorders like chronic fatigue syndrome.[27]

The use of healthcare services is also largely sprung by unemployment and increasing rate of poverty. Even though some government programs and assistance is available, benefits vary considerably from place to place and are continually being reevaluated.[28] A person who is unemployed due to CFS is affected by this type of problem. Although unforeseen circumstances arise, there are also admirable changes that are improving hospital care around the world, such as advanced technologies that allow for more accurate diagnosis and more appropriate treatment.[29] For CFS patients to receive proper and adequate treatment, a hospital must increase the quality of its health care primarily by responding to and rectifying organizational problems. Quality health care equates to the apt management of hospital patients, together with properly educated staff who can respond to miscellaneous cases. As a general conclusion, of course, the proper management of these issues leads to better treatment of the patients, especially CFS sufferers, in a hospital system.[30]

In a study in 2001, scientists determined that there were a significant number of CFS patients unsatisfied not only with the quality of health care delivery, but also with the interpersonal skills possessed by their attending physician.[31] In the research that they conducted, sixty-eight patients completed a survey about their overall satisfaction with the medical assistance that they received since the onset of their condition and their perspective on certain aspects of health care. Two-thirds of the patients were disappointed in the quality of medical care that they received. Those patients who were dissatisfied significantly (a) were more likely to protest about the delay, contradictions, or misunderstandings regarding their diagnosis, (b) received and simultaneously rejected a psychiatric diagnosis, or (c) saw doctors as indifferent, doubtful, or uninformed about CFS. They also distrusted the advice given to them since they saw it as both insufficient and conflicting in nature.[32]

Those patients who were satisfied were pointedly more likely to distinguish their doctors as considerate, supportive, and committed to uncovering their illness. These patients also claimed that they didn't expect their doctors to cure CFS and perceived their general physicians as the source of their greatest help in the course of their illness. Many patients were also critical of the small number of treatments employed, although this matter wasn't a great factor affecting their general satisfaction.[33] This study revealed that a doctor who has more information about the illness is preferred. Since the patient is already knowledge-able that his illness has no particular cure, he prefers someone with whom he can talk informatively and communicate on a much more personal level.

The findings of this study then alluded that hospital care was evaluated by CFS patients less on the doctor's ability to cure their illness but rather on his interpersonal skills and knowledge about the illness.[34] This then would be greatly affected by the uneven distribution of the health workforce around the world, such as in Africa, where thirty-six out of fifty-seven countries are currently facing a shortage in human resources, leaving fewer adequately informed health personnel to address the needs of CFS patients.[35] The authors and their study have advocated better communication and better education for hospital physicians in the diagnosis and management of CFS. Generally, the outcome of CFS patients' treatment has its foundation in the ability of healthcare personnel to cater to their physical, psychological, and interpersonal needs.

Doctor Involvement in CFS Hospital Care

The physician is responsible for the medical diagnosis and for shaping the therapy required by a person suffering with chronic fatigue syndrome. The physician's role has traditionally been the treatment of disease and trauma; however, many hospital doctors are now including health promotion as well as disease prevention in their repertoire.[36]

In the hospital care of CFS patients, doctors carry on with diagnosis, treatment, and proper communication with their patients. Their primary obligation is to correctly diagnose the patient's health situation as well as to provide them proper information on what to do, what they should expect, and what they may experience throughout the course of their illness. Although CFS patients prefer a more personal relationship with their doctor, hospital-based healthcare professionals must also be straightforward and precise with the information they share, even if it's bad news for the client.[37]

The attending physician is adequately informed about the disorder and is capable of giving the proper treatment to the patient suffering from CFS. Most likely, physicians who treat chronic fatigue must focus on treating multiple symptoms that prevail during the course of the condition. These two primary symptoms are sleep abnormalities and chronic pain. The treatment of both greatly helps the recovery of the patient. Proper sleep management helps the CFS patient regain strength and makes him more relaxed despite the cyclical stints of fatigue. Healing the chronic pain also helps improve the CFS client's living situation at the hospital, and the reduction of the pain provides more comfort and thus enhanced health.[38]

Hospital physicians are responsible for monitoring the patient's daily activities and for finding suitable treatments. At times, patients misinterpret the meaning of exercise and physical activity, but for a physician attending a CFS patient, minimal exercise is required, depending on the severity of the case. The goal is to help the hospital patient regain mobility gradually by practicing normal bodily movements. Of course, the severity of the condition must be accurately diagnosed in order for the hospital to determine the extent of appropriate activities for the patient. Basically, the physician is there to guide and instruct the patient and to ensure that he systematically follows advices for his recovery.[39]

Psychologically, physicians aid in the recovery of CFS through interpersonal communication, since CFS patients may suffer mental disarray due to the loss of their jobs, their inability to perform daily tasks, and the like. Physicians become more of a trusted friend than a doctor. Knowing that there's someone else who can properly empathize with this condition and who can give credible advice can help frustrated individuals who are suffering from CFS.[40]

ANALYSIS

Undoubtedly, the involvement of a physician in the hospital care of a CFS patient is vital. Since a one-stop cure for this disorder is yet to be found, treatments can only manage the patient's symptoms. The hospital's help in determining the appropriate course of treatment for the patient is paramount. Whether it's the management of stress, sleep, or daily activities or prescribing medications, the role of the hospital has always been to give proper diagnosis and to ensure that the patient recovers from the symptoms of CFS.

Part III

Many Faces

8

FATIGUE AND THE HUMAN BODY

Fatigue, generally expressed as the deterioration of physical perfor-mance, is a complex physical phenomenon that affects both the physio-logical and psychological disposition and functioning of the human body.[1] It's likened to a feeling of tiredness and exhaustion, a state wherein the individual lacks vitality, alertness, and motivation (subjec-tive fatigue); is unable to accomplish tasks with expected quality and timeliness (objective fatigue); and exhibits significant changes in physio-logical processes, such as sustained muscular contractions (physiological fatigue).[2]

It can be caused by (a) motor units, such as muscle contractions (peripheral fatigue) or (b) bustles in the brain or the spine (central fatigue). Fatigue may be the result of overwork, lack of curative sleep, anxiety, boredom, or lack of exercise. It can also be a symptom caused by illness, medication, medical treatment, anxiety, and depression. It can be an accumulation of fatigue-causing stress or an acute application of significant stress that leads to a *failing point*, thereby triggering the brain to take impulsive action such as daytime dozing.[3]

Fresh developments in understanding fatigue have also led to de-cryption of CFS occurrences, also known as myalgic encephalomyelitis, which has proven to be as serious as other common chronic illnesses. Fatigue is even considered to be more blighting, such that patients with those illnesses associated with CFS (usually heart failure, suicide, and cancer) die relatively younger. Fatigue weighs on significant anatomical perturbations (i.e., nervous, endocrine, circulatory), but exhibits external symptoms that may not always indicate serious health concerns. A disadvantage, however, is the perception of CFS: whether it deserves the same attention as those with other common chronic ailments like heart disease and cancer. The disadvantage affects the societal construct and perception of CFS, where the possibilities of patient recovery lie: patients report poor experiences with healthcare providers, some of whom doubt the validity of CFS as a real medical problem.[4]

While the signals of fatigue on the organs can be identified by specific archetypes such as respiration, heartbeat, skin temperature, sweating, and pulse rate, the effect of fatigue can be observed from how the CFS patient's vital organs react to the stress stimulus that causes it, aside from the perceived disposition of the individual (i.e., psychological bearing of fatigue).[5]

Based on various studies that have pointed out the different effects of fatigue on the human body, the influence of fatigue can be focused on six anatomical systems: the nervous system, the endocrine system, the respiratory system, the circulatory system, the musculoskeletal system, and the digestive system.[6] Each system has its own story about how tiredness becomes a threat to the normal functions of the body, as well as how these threats are treated to prevent possible dangers. That said, the rest of this chapter describes the effects of fatigue on these six human body systems based on contemporary findings from various fields.

FATIGUE AND THE NERVOUS AND ENDOCRINE SYSTEMS

Nervous System

Although fatigue is usually associated with the exertion of muscular effort, it's possible to experience fatigue without physical activity, that is, while performing normal daily activities, during postoperative recovery, and when confronting sleep disturbances or deprivation. Fatigue that occurs in this way may be attributed to mechanisms in the central nervous system (CNS), which may later be expressed physically as the following:

- Underperformance;
- Decreased motivation;
- Lethargy;
- Tiredness;
- Loss of motor coordination;
- Obvious confusion and disorientation;
- Loss of concentration;
- Difficulty in processing and categorizing information;
- Hardship in remembering words or phrases; and
- Sensory disorientation.

A person suffering from fatigue may also experience sensory overload, such as hypersensitivity to light and sound, and emotional overload, which may cause anxiety attacks. This is known as CNS fatigue or neuromuscular fatigue. Unlike muscular fatigue, CNS fatigue is triggered by activities in the brain and the spinal column, which can occur even without immediate observable stress.[7]

Understanding CNS fatigue entails knowing how the central nervous system works. Studies in 1997 and 2001 explain that full fatigue occurs during increased levels of serotonin (also known as hydroxytryptamine [5-HT]) and lower levels of dopamine in the brain.[8] The mushrooming levels of serotonin are caused by an increase in free tryptophan (TRP) in the brain, which is later synthesized into serotonin.

The TRP is usually connected with albumin in the blood and is transported to the brain via specific receptors, which the TRP shares with branched-chain amino acid (BCAA). However, during exercise, fatty acids separate the TRP from their connection with the albumin, while the BCAA is molded into energy, thus leaving the TRP free to connect with the receptors and cross through the blood-brain barrier. This causes the increase of TRP in the brain, and eventually an elevation in serotonin levels. Given this process, serotonin levels may swell in the brain when fatty acids are abundant and the BCAA is low; this will subsequently increase fatigue.[9]

Although this usually occurs during exercise, there is evidence that the level of serotonin can climb even during a sedentary state, when experiencing immobilizing stress (caused by the redoubled movement of TRP to the brain), or when consuming food rich in carbohydrates without exercising. High levels of serotonin are also observed in elderly people, individuals who are depressed, and those with liver failure, renal disease, and appetite disorders. [10]

Several theories of CNS fatigue have been conjectured throughout the years. These may be categorized into physiological and psychological treatments: physiological implications are nutrition, medication, and hormonal supplements. Some studies have found that the introduction of BCAA can reduce the potential for CNS fatigue, especially for those doing exercises. Psychological treatments include rest and meditation. However, the most common advice in addressing CNS fatigue is moderation in activities: avoiding both a sedentary lifestyle and the overexertion of muscles. [11]

Endocrine System

Endocrine-related fatigue is a reduction in physiological and psychological capacity, usually associated with an ailment of the endocrine system. This is difficult to diagnose because oftentimes it is overshadowed by some other ailment or dismissed as psychological in nature. Tests, unless directed to determine fatigue, don't necessarily point in this direction; endocrine tests tend to show normal results. As a consequence, fatigue remains untreated. [12]

Endocrine-provoked fatigue differs from other causes because in addition to fatigue indicators (i.e., retardation of movement, confusion, and weakness or tiredness), patients experience a variety of symptoms. They can include the following:

- Irregular menstrual period;
- Abnormal body hair growth (for women);
- Carbohydrate craving;
- Sleep disturbances or deprivation;
- Depression;
- Dizziness when standing;
- Concentration problems;
- Unexplained weight loss or weight gain;
- Osteoporosis;
- Breast discharge;
- Memory loss;
- Decreased sex drive; and

- Erectile problems.

This is expected in endocrine-related fatigue and is connected with marked disorders such as the following:

- Thyroid disease;
- Growth hormone deficiency;
- Adrenal insufficiency;
- Metabolic syndrome (also known as insulin resistance);
- Diabetes;
- Low glucose sugar;
- Cushing's syndrome;
- Deficiencies in androgen;
- Vitamin D; and
- Estrogen.

If the fatigue symptoms persist and recur for more than six months and notably affect the patient's performance, a CFS diagnosis is strongly considered, which requires a different set of protocols for treatment. Treatment of endocrine-caused fatigue requires two important points. First is diagnosis. As stated earlier, fatigue caused by dysfunctions in the endocrine system is diagnosed only in consultation with an endocrinologist who administers tests specifically to identify the cause of the fatigue.[13]

Proper diagnosis enables medical practitioners as well as affected persons to determine proper treatment. Treatment occurring in unison with comorbid illness comes second. Fatigue, if associated with an existing ailment, such as diabetes and adult growth hormone deficiency, needs to be addressed as soon as possible. Hence, treatment of the fatigue as a symptom calls for the treatment of the whole ailment as well.[14]

FATIGUE AND THE RESPIRATORY AND CIRCULATORY SYSTEMS

Respiratory System

Respiratory muscle fatigue is the inability of the respiratory muscles to generate enough pressure to maintain proper ventilation during respiration, which can eventually result in *ventilatory failure*. This is usually caused by lung diseases, wherein the respiratory system suffers from added stress from an ailment.[15]

The mechanisms for respiratory muscular fatigue and muscle fatigue are similar: that is, the brain signals the muscles to exert effort (or contract) in order to undertake a target action. What differs about normal muscle fatigue and respiratory muscle fatigue is the unmistakeable interaction between central and peripheral fatigue. Both central and peripheral fatigue is observed in respiratory muscular fatigue. Studies have shown an equal decrease in effort from the brain and respiratory muscles during episodes of fatigue.[16]

The relationships among the body's systems are interdependent, such that an emergency mechanism is engaged when extreme fatigue occurs. To illustrate, imagine that a CFS patient's lung muscles are already fatigued, meaning that they can no longer sustain the pressure or load they bear. In order to protect the lung muscles from totally collapsing, the brain ceases sending activation signals to the muscles, which in turn disables the respiratory muscles from exerting further stress to the already fatigued area. This will therefore delay respiratory fatigue from occurring, and respiratory failure is stalled. This happens as a protective mechanism of the CNS, adapting against possible damages to the respiratory muscles. Otherwise, the unceasing signal from the brain for muscles to exert more effort could lead to irreparable respiratory failure and eventually significantly compromise the person's health.[17]

Respiratory muscular fatigue can be treated in two ways: (1) decreasing the demand on the lung muscles and (2) improving the endurance of lung muscles. Regarding the first note, it's logical that respiratory muscular fatigue can be addressed by reducing the need for lung muscles to exert energy. This can be done by reducing the resistance in the lung muscles. As for the second point, improving the strength of lung muscles is necessary to ensure the endurance of the lungs. This can be done through medication, training, rest, and proper nutrition.[18]

Circulatory System

As the brain is important in delivering instruction for action to the different parts of the body, so too is the circulatory system, which serves as a pathway for oxygen, vital nutrients, and hormones to ensure the efficient functioning of the CFS sufferer's organs. Persons with cardio-vascular fatigue exhibit symptoms of orthostatic intolerance (i.e., the inability to stay upright). Simply put, when a CFS sufferer experiences poor blood circulation, the different organs of the body have a hard time carrying out their regular functions and duties. The circulatory system, constituting the heart, blood, arteries, and veins, functions as the oxygen and nutrient carrier to the different organs of the body.[19]

If the circulatory system is unable to deliver the essentials for normal body function, the inability is probably due to a malfunctioning auto-nomic nervous system, and therefore the CFS patient starts to experi-ence muscle cramping. *Hypotension* is accompanied by dizziness and light-headedness, visual disturbances, and slow response to stimuli. Postural orthostatic tachycardia syndrome (an increase in heart rate and a drop in pulse upon standing) or delayed postural hypotension (symp-toms of hypotension occurring minutes after standing up) can also strike.[20]

To determine the presence of stress or fatigue in the circulatory system and specifically in the heart, a tilt test is usually administered to patients who exhibit a fleeting increase in heart rate together with a brusque decrease in blood pressure when standing up (that quickly improves after sitting or lying down). Monitoring for *arrhythmia* is also undertaken to determine regularity of heartbeat.[21] First-line treatment for a person experiencing cardiovascular fatigue would be to drink much water and take in a bit more salt. Movement (avoiding a seden-tary state) is necessary to assist blood circulation. Patients are also ad-vised to wear medical stockings that'll help in blood circulation.[22]

FATIGUE AND THE MUSCULOSKELETAL AND DIGESTIVE SYSTEMS

Musculoskeletal System

Musculoskeletal fatigue occurs when muscles or joints have limited function. This occurs when muscles are unable to generate sufficient force for and velocity of the contractions needed to achieve an activity.[23] Muscular fatigue originates in either the muscles or joints. Either way, such a form of fatigue is usually exhibited by hindrance in movement, inability to exert normal levels of strength for a task, and an overall collapse while performing a task. The musculoskeletal system can normally recover from fatigue after sufficient rest, in contrast to CFS-related fatigue wherein the muscle is unable to recuperate even with rest.

The delivery of a message from the brain to the muscle can be summarized in three stages: (1) the central motor unit delivers the message to the target muscle, (2) enzymes are metabolized to produce energy for the action, and (3) the muscles are excited, which leads to contraction or application of force. The message contains what sort of activity is to be conducted and how much energy is needed.[24]

Muscle fatigue occurs when the amount of energy required is greater than the amount of energy the body can provide and when there are disruptions in the transmission from the neuromuscular transmission to the *actin-myosin cross bridging*. The energy requirement, however, is determined not only at the peripheral level (the degree to which a muscle group can contract), but also on the neural level. Based on that, it can be noted that muscle fatigue can happen at any time during the process of determining the required physical effort (central fatigue) to the actual exertion of effort or contraction of muscles to complete the activity (peripheral fatigue).[25]

Digestive System

Digestive system fatigue is caused by the overuse of energy to digest food. In the digestive system, whose operations are affected by the autonomic nervous system, fatigue in the generally happens when there's food intolerance or when the person is suffering from Hirschprung disease, *achalasia cardia, cancer cachexia*, and sphincter abnormalities. Essentially, digestion-related fatigue is caused by issues in food processing: when the routine of digesting food is disrupted due to other issues, the body exerts more energy to cope with the digestion requirements.[26]

This overexertion of effort comes with gastrointestinal discomforts such as diarrhea, constipation, or alternating diarrhea and constipation, abdominal cramps, bloating, nausea, and anorexia. If digestive troubles persist, the absorption of essential nutrients may not take place, affecting the rest of the organs, consequently causing more fatigue. Suggestions to address digestion-related fatigue include avoiding foods that exacerbate the CFS patient's condition, abstaining from processed foods, and thoroughly chewing food.[27]

ANALYSIS

Although fatigue might appear to be a mere symptom signaling the need for rest, the concept of fatigue has garnered significant interest from various fields due to its impact on a person's well-being. In surgery, for instance, a high rate of errors in medical treatment that may be attributed to fatigue and sleep deprivation has led to calls for change in healthcare protocols.[28]

The sports industry has invested significant funds in the development of training programs to help to prevent muscular fatigue and its effects on athletic performance. Automobile regulatory boards have undertaken tremendous efforts to institutionalize road safety measures to counter possible effects of fatigued driving. Even long-term treatments such as those for cancer have established protocols for addressing fatigue-related reactions to ailments and treatments. Studies on treating fatigue, medical or otherwise, became a running objective for various professional turfs, but fatigue still eludes complete understanding.

9

VIRAL, NEUROPSYCHIATRIC, AND NEUROENDOCRINE HYPOTHESES

Viruses' structures and reproduction strategies are diverse. The virus is usually rather small and it replicates in many ways. Even a small quantity of virus particles can affect a person's heath. Still, viruses don't carry out metabolic processes, and there are restricted *intracellular* parasites that are inanimate. Viruses represent the class of capsid-encoding organisms, or CEOs.

VIRAL HYPOTHESIS FOR CHRONIC FATIGUE SYNDROME

There are three primary hypotheses for chronic fatigue syndrome (CFS): the progressive hypothesis, the regressive hypothesis, and the virus-first hypothesis. The progressive or escape hypothesis posits that viruses originate from genetic elements that obtained the capacity to progress between cells. Regressive or reductive hypotheses declare that a virus is a remnant of cellular organisms, and the virus-first hypothesis claims that viruses predate and coevolved with current cellular hosts.[1]

Retroviruses are viruses that through progressive biological processes become infectious agents. Large DNA viruses take a regressive course, by which a once-independent body lost its key genes over a point of time and took up a parasitic reproduction strategy. Viruses may arise several times through several bodily processes. Continuous research in areas like genomics, structural biology, and microbiology may supply answers yet to be discovered, but until now no precise explanation about the origin of viruses exists.[2]

Using the aforesaid pathways, an active viral infection that's often bracketed with the symptoms of CFS has guided researchers to hypothesize that viruses stimulate the syndrome. The hormone, immune, and central nervous systems and the possibility that stress, reproduction, or reactivation of latent viruses could adjust to the immune system to cause CFS should be explored.[3]

Vagus Nerve Infection

The vagus nerve infection hypothesis (VNIH), suggests that nerve-loving viruses cause an immune response that's difficult to detect, sparking fatigue and other prognostic symptoms of CFS.[4] This hypothesis suggests that infections cause CFS and that the most significant thing about the infection is its source, which is the vagus nerve, the largest in the body. This wandering nerve stretches over the human trunk, conveying its roots into most organs of the body. An infection doesn't need to be powerful; it need only be present in the vagus nerve to generate havoc in the brain.[5]

As the vagus nerve winds through the body, it approaches viral havens that harbor herpesviruses such as the cytomegalovirus and Epstein-Barr virus. Nearly all humans bear some of these herpesviruses in latent form; biological events or stressors permit reactivation. Upon recrudescence, it's thought that these viruses leave the nerves and run into glial cells that try to gobble them up. The glial cells put out all manner of nerve-exciting and pro-inflammatory compounds in the presence of viruses. The vagus nerve receptors sniff out the alarm signals and inform the brain that an infection exists, and it'll send out signals to shut off or slow down the movements of the CFS patient's torso.[6]

New Model of Fatigue

Studies on animals show that fatigue and flulike symptoms thrive when the vagus nerve is infected.[7] Flulike symptoms that are attendant with infections may not survive without the vagus nerve, because rodents infected with pathogens don't act sick after having their vagus nerves cut. The symptoms of a sickness would be intense and uncontrollable if the vagus nerve receptors were endlessly attacked with these cytokines. A raging infection can have a similar allergic response in the vagus nerve when glial cells encircle the nerve. Researchers propose that CFS could in fact be a hodgepodge of glial cell diseases.[8]

Infections That Don't Appear in the Blood

Researchers aren't able to detect these groups of viruses through biopsy of the vagus nerve and in the blood because the viruses may be expanding their path of destruction onto different tissues. Studies have been performed using HIV protein to mimic a certain nervous system infection.[9] Researchers discovered that glial cells stack up and begin to raise pro-inflammatory cytokines to handle the intruder. However, cytokines couldn't be found in the rodents' bloodstreams even though the animal acted sick, isolated, and despondent. Proof of growth in cytokine levels was attainable only when the rodent's spinal cord was sampled near the infected region.[10]

Cytokines may be found in the spinal fluid when the vagus nerve is infected close to the brain stem but they wouldn't be traceable in the blood. However, cytokines reside in the blood and not in the spinal fluid when the vagus nerve is infected in the abdominal region. Cytokines, for example, are revealed if the lungs of the mice with lung infections were sampled. It's therefore believed that cytokines can't be distinguished at all, wherever the infection may be.[11]

Animal studies have been proposed to improve the understanding of vagus nerve infections. Magnetic resonance imaging might have the capacity to identify viral lesions in the cardinal nervous system tissues, and special PET scans may be used to evaluate microglial activation. Moreover, reports on seriously ill patients and cadaver studies should be carried out in the future to discover viral infections, activated glia, and inflammation.[12]

Neuropsychiatric Hypothesis for Chronic Fatigue Syndrome

Neuropsychiatric problems are far-flung in chronic fatigue syndrome and are connected to disorders of behavior and mood. Depression and major depressive disorder (MDD) are often experienced by CFS patients. The exact causal link between CFS and MDD is still not understood, despite much research, resulting in the development of polarized hypotheses concerning the true clinical causes of CFS.[13]

A number of intriguing immunological and inflammatory clarifications have recently been revealed, proposing that CFS and MDD are recognizably different yet have related conditions. The overlap between CFS and MDD is the shared inflammatory, oxidative, and nitrosative stress (IO&NS) pathways. Chronic fatigue syndrome is also linked to neuropsychological symptoms such as impaired memory, attention, and response time. The syndrome is a systemic, severe, obtained illness of extreme fatigue that can't be moderated by rest and might even be worsened by neuropsychiatric and physical activity.[14]

Neuropsychiatric Features

Chronic fatigue syndrome sufferers often describe a variety of neuropsychiatric symptoms, typically marked by a decrease in cognitive functions. Until now, neuropsychological research in chronic fatigue syndrome has strived to envision the exact identity of cognitive complaints in CFS. Objective proof of cognitive distraction has been connected to a deficiency in reaction time, with memory and attention being the most knotty for patients who have CFS.[15]

Written reports have revealed a substantial connection between depressive, somatoform, anxiety, and personality-associated disorders and CFS. Many CFS patients are whispered to be suffering from psychiatric disorders, particularly depressive illness, and studies indicate remarkable comorbidity between depression and CFS. Fifteen to 40 percent of its patients were judged to be suffering from major depression, 5 to 15 percent of patients were estimated to have somatization disorders, and 20 percent of its patients have been found with anxiety disorders. Nevertheless, the huge majority of neuropsychiatric information is committed to depression because depression is one of the most important clinical obstacles faced in CFS.[16]

Depressive Illness

Depression shares several remarkable overlapping symptoms with CFS, and some of its eminent characteristics are poor concentration, memory difficulties, sleep disturbance, and overwhelming fatigue. The exact relationship between depression and CFS remains unknown, and this is still an area of intense disagreement. The chief arenas that the debate centers on are: (a) disabilities inflicted by the disease activity, (b) that depression and CFS share sources, and (c) that CFS is actually considered a configuration of depression.[17]

Although absence of a confirmed cause of CFS has created a rift in the debate and steered several researchers to claim that CFS has psychiatric roots, CFS is recognized as a disabling disorder with astronomical rates of depression. The magnitude of depression in CFS is significantly more conspicuous than those revealed in other chronic maladies.[18]

Investigating Major Depressive Disorder

Major depressive disorder is a neuropsychiatric disorder characterized by pathologically impaired sleep, depressed mood, tiredness, and ephemeral motivation. Major depressive disorder (MDD) and CFS symptoms overlap astonishingly, thus CFS literature specifies that MDD is the single most prevalent psychiatric illness linked with CFS. Yet, not all CFS patients encounter psychiatric symptoms, therefore it's sensible to state that even though MDD is an important characteristic of CFS, it affects some but not all, CFS sufferers.[19]

In terms of symptom grouping, major depressive disorder and CFS are categorized differently. The Beck depression inventory (BDI) differentiates patients with CFS from those with MDD, and this study discloses that MDD patients are recognized by symptoms such as self-reproach and disturbed mood, while CFS patients had BDI scores associated particularly with symptoms of fatigue and physical complaints.[20]

Compared with MDD patients, CFS patients show less difficulty with guilt, suicidal ideation, and self-esteem. The MDD patients also have "inward attribution" of their symptoms, whereas CFS clients were prone to blame their symptoms on physical sources. Recently, it's been discovered that in order to successfully distinguish between those suffering from MDD and CFS, one needs to consider the severity of shortness of breath, unrefreshing sleep, impaired concentration, and post-exercise malaise.[21]

These analyses illustrate that even though CFS and MDD share numerous similar symptoms, such as poor concentration, pain, sleep disruption, and profound fatigue, CFS and MDD are distinct ill-nesses.[22] The analyses also emphasize that the kind of symptoms indi-cated by CFS patients are dissimilar. By observing their reaction to physical exertion, CFS patients could be differentiated from depressive patients.[23] After exertion, CFS patients experience increased fatigue, whereas the depressed patients enjoy a rise in positive mood. In short, experts determined that typical CFS symptoms like sore throat, painful lymph nodes, and post-exertional malaise aren't commonly noticed in MDD, because the latter disorder points to a separate underpinning of disease.[24]

Biological Foundation of Major Depressive Disorder

The connection between CFS and MDD is multifarious, yet, in spite of the complexities, there's visible proof that the connection between the two may be distinguished through the IO&NS pathways. This pathway introduces a complex series of biochemical responses that results in the destruction of free radicals and nitric oxide outcomes at a cellular lev-el.[25] In research, IO&NS was discovered to be accountable for destroy-ing fatty acids, proteins, and DNA and was remarkably connected to patients' complaints of flulike malaise, fatigue, and muscle pain.[26]

The stimulation of IO&NS pathways is recognized to increase fa-tigue and body symptoms, and it could be triggered by immune disor-ders, infections, and psychosocial stress.[27] This shows that CFS and MDD might share clinical symptoms of a shared IO&NS pathway, but it's also been claimed that CFS and MDD could be differentiated from each other by concentrating on research that appears from other biolog-ical systems.[28] For instance, MDD is traditionally linked with elevated cortisol levels and increased hypothalamus-pituitary-adrenal (HPA) axis process.[29]

Raised cortisol in MDD produces difficulties in executive thought functioning, visuo-spatial memory, and verbal memory, but HPA ex-periments on CFS patients discovered lesser, not higher, cortisol lev-els.[30] The damaged HPA axis operation is believed to be accountable for the symptoms of headaches, post-exertional malaise, and tiredness in CFS sufferers, unlike for MDD.[31]

Currently the *adrenal androgens dehydroepiandrosterone (DHEA)* and *dehydroepiandrosterone-sulphate (DHEA-S)* are the center of attention, though less intensively studied in reference to CFS. The metabolic connection between DHEA and cortisol is an intense area of interest because in order to preserve homeostasis, the production of androgens transfer to glucocorticoids throughout physical and psychological stress.[32] Nevertheless, in an initial research of DHEA in CFS, scientists found that the predicted metabolic transfer from HDEA to cortisol didn't occur in CFS patients.[33]

The research also emphasized that CFS patients displayed lower levels of DHEA and remarkably lesser DHEA-S in contrast to MDD patients and healthy controls. Furthermore, patients reacted positively to DHEA replacement treatment in a small uncontrolled test.[34]

Depression and Illness Limitations

Since CFS is linked with serious illness-imposed limitations, it has caused some researchers to declare that depressive illness in CFS is merely a natural reaction to the debilitating symptoms encountered by its sufferers. There was no cogent proof that patients with CFS are really *hypochondriacal*, hence psychiatric illness is concluded to be an outcome of CFS rather than something that caused the development of the syndrome.[35]

In research comparing patients with CFS and patients with MDD and multiple sclerosis (MS), it was discovered that patients with CFS resembled the MS patients more closely than the MDD group, and the study also noted that the CFS group encountered fewer *axis 1 disorders* than MDD patients.[36]

Generalized Anxiety Disorder

Anxiety disorder involves reactive stress due to medical conditions or substances, post-traumatic stress disorder, agoraphobia, social anxiety, generalized anxiety, panic disorder, and other trauma-related reactions. The primary characteristic of anxiety disorder is mental or physical anxiety that is out of proportion with the recent condition and that particularly affects the quality or functioning of life. People with CFS were found to have higher rates of generalized anxiety disorder (GAD), which was placed by an earlier beginning and high rates of psychiatric comorbidity that specifies a tendency to develop CFS.[37]

Nevertheless, there's no clear understanding about the specific neurobiological changes that lead to this condition, although generalized anxiety disorder is a regular and significant disorder. Even though some research to date has been performed on neurobiological function in GAD patients, only limited qualified data is available for depression. The bridges between CFS and GAD, such as sleep abnormalities, sympathetic hyperactivity, and vegetated cerebral blood flow, still require more analysis.[38]

Somatoform Disorder

Somatization is described as the tendency to convert psychological distress into physical symptoms and obtain medical assistance to reduce them.[39] Somatization encompasses a wide scope of patients' perceptions and experiences, which results in patients reporting symptoms that are completely physical.[40] It's usual to assume that clinically unknown patient complaints are the result of underlying emotional distress among these three groups of somatization behavior.

In that respect, somatization disorder is also a recognized psychiatric barrier in the *Diagnostic and Statistical Manual of Mental Disorders 3 (DSM-III)*. Somatization disorder is diagnosed when an individual suffers at least thirteen of its thirty-five recognized symptoms over a period of years, with onset before the age of thirty.[41] Surveys of psychiatric illness in CFS have demonstrated extremely high rates of somatization disorders, and in other analyses, investigators discovered that patients displayed a higher rate of somatization disorder symptoms than in clients with multiple sclerosis.[42] The research, however, specifies that few of the patients with CFS represent the precise DSM-III-R standard for somatization disorder.

Further research disclosed that changing how somatization symptoms were categorized also changed the likelihood of diagnosis of somatization disorder.[43] An example of changing the attribution of somatization symptoms would be to code the CFS symptoms as psychiatric. It was discovered that six of thirty patients exhibited a lifetime history of major depression when symptoms attributed to CFS were abolished.[44]

However, twelve of thirty patients described a lifetime history of major depressive illness as diagnostic protocols of all symptoms were used. These studies thus displayed that the recognition of CFS relies upon a patient's account of physical symptoms and the researcher's conclusion that there's no physical cause for the symptoms. Lastly, if CFS patients were covering up their psychological sufferings with physical symptoms, then there should be a reverse connection between anxiety and depression symptoms and the reported numbers of physical symptoms.[45] Yet CFS patients haven't detailed anxiety-related, depressive, and physical symptoms simultaneously.[46]

Personality Disorder

Evidence from research specifies that personality disorder—mainly obsessive-compulsive disorder (OCD)—exists in approximately 40 percent of CFS patients.[47] In research, 37 percent of CFS cases met the criterion for at least one personality disorder such as borderline or histrionic personality disorder.[48] Among CFS patients, there are higher rates of personality disorder compared to nonpatients. Furthermore, a few of the measures applied could increase the probability of finding personality disorder in patients who are chronically ill. In one study, comorbid depression was reported as personality pathologies.[49]

Reaction Time

Numerous neuropsychological inquiries have evaluated and analyzed the reaction time of patients with CFS, based on easy and complex information-processing assignments. The most noted cognitive difficulty discovered in CFS relates to an abnormality in patient information-processing efficiency and speed.[50] Countless research indicates that patients with CFS don't perform well on coursework that requires swift handling of information and on time-limited and complex assignments.[51] Currently, in a population-based analysis of neuropsychological performance, it was learned that in contrast to controls, patients with CFS displayed a remarkable decrease in motor speed.[52]

Furthermore, CFS patients with higher levels of cognitive difficulties also displayed more immune abnormalities, which suggests that cognitive difficulties in CFS can be described independently of those that generally exist with depression.[53] Lastly, the cognitive dysfunction seen in CFS patients is unlikely to be explained by anxiety and depression.[54] These analyses specify that CFS patients display moderate to significant abnormalities in reaction times, and the information-processing difficulties of CFS patients contribute to abnormalities in reaction-time assignments.[55] Fine motor speed was not lost in individuals with CFS. Thus, it's unlikely that motor performance is primarily connected to slower reaction times.[56]

Memory

Scientific opinion about links between memory problems and CFS is split; some research found proof of memory deficits in CFS while others didn't.[57] This conflict is linked to nonverbal and verbal memory problems in CFS sufferers.[58] Most neuropsychological research on memory in CFS utilized visual and verbal memory tests. Specifically, some trials evaluated memory utilizing word lists, and in terms of verbal memory, some analyses indicate minimal "word list" learning.[59] Recognition, delayed recall, and immediate recollection were abnormal in CFS cases. Patients with CFS have trouble with obtaining verbal information and require greater effort in memorizing a word list compared to healthy controls.[60] The conclusion was that the memory burdens encountered by CFS patients are connected to compromises in their ability to recall verbal information. These memory difficulties may be a result of poor initial learning.[61] An analysis of patients with MDD and CFS and healthy controls discovered that patients with CFS show deviant brain physiology.[62]

Attention

The scientific research models about working memory and attention span maintain that they're both essential cognitive functions for productive learning and reasoning. In a functional MRI study of the working memory, significant differences were discovered in the brain activation between control subjects and CFS patients, especially as demands were increased on the working memory.[63] The inquiry concluded that patients with CFS didn't engage working memory in a similar manner as healthy subjects, and the outcome specifies that the CFS patients had to use additional approaches to neutralize their underlying cognitive difficulties. In research with patients focusing over extended periods of time, CFS sufferers also showed consistent difficulty with working memory.[64]

NEUROENDOCRINE HYPOTHESIS FOR CHRONIC FATIGUE SYNDROME

The neuroendocrine system consists of the nervous and the endocrine systems, which work together to keep the body functioning regularly. The nervous system and the endocrine system consist of neuroendocrine cells, which are situated throughout the body and release hormones transmitting messages to cells. The interactions between the brain and the glands that produce hormones could assist in explaining the neuroendocrine symptoms of CFS. Thought-provoking studies have proposed a neuroendocrine context for CFS, but the true vices these symptoms carry out are still enigmas. Scientists have discovered that several patients with CFS have low levels of cortisol, which is a hormone processed by the HPA axis that holds the potential key to fatigue and sleep disorders. Neuroendocrine participation in CFS and its treatment strategies to enhance a patient's daily life still require further research from quite a few fields of study.[65]

Disturbed Neuroendocrine-Immune Interactions

The symptomatology in CFS was hypothesized to be an effect from abnormalities in inter-organ transmission rather than from oddities in a specific organ system. A feature of inter-organ transmission is the reactivity of certain receptors in the target organs as well as the production and secretion of mediator chemicals by other organ systems. Hence, variations in the way target organs react to the mediators and changes in the actual level of neuroendocrine mediators might result in poor transmission. Poor transmission could lead to the pathophysiology of CFS and might explain the mixed outcomes cited in many works that concentrate on a specific organ system. Currently, the neuroendocrine system and the immune system have been well proven to closely interact with each other.[66]

Psychological stress is applied to modulate immune reactivity through complex interactions that utilize the autonomic nervous system as well as the HPA axis while the immune system cells express receptors for neurotransmitters and hormones. Activating these receptors results in modulation of immune responsiveness. The immune system cells that are easily attainable in the peripheral blood and that could be examined *ex vivo* are used to inspect the integrity of neuroendocrine regulation. To date, the pathophysiology of CFS is still poorly understood, and analysis performed over the past ten years indicates that the syndrome can't be identified by a deficiency in one specific organ system. Current perspectives are therefore not meant to define changes in a single system, but to inspect the integrity of inter-organ transmission in CFS patients.[67]

In a study of inter-organ transmission, the interaction between the neuroendocrine system and the immune system was chosen as a model system. The outcome reveals that the transmission between the neuroendocrine system and the immune system is different for adolescents than it is for adults. It was also hypothesized that neuroendocrine-immune transmission abnormalities in chronic fatigue syndrome are a result of preexisting psychological distress and precipitating events such as viral infections. In summary, the recent analysis reveals that chemical exchange between neuroendocrine mediators and the immune system is disturbed in CFS.[68]

Critical Issues of the Neuroendocrine System

The basic HPA role in CFS still requires clarification, and there's proof that the HPA axis malfunctions in patients with CFS, even though experimentation has produced inconsistent outcomes. Neuroendocrine faults, CFS, cytokine abnormalities, and orthostatic intolerance may be interconnected. Cytokines, which are chemical messengers, activate the HPA axis each time a body is experiencing an infection or is under stress. Interleukin-6 (IL-6), tumor necrosis factor (TNF), and a few others have been implicated in CFS.[69]

Research has revealed that corticotrophin-releasing hormone (CRH) levels in a human's cerebrospinal fluid is normal or low in patients with CFS but might increase in depressed patients.[70] Patients with CFS also display a decreased cortisol reaction when compared to patients with depression. Even though there was no correlation between CFS and stress, stressors such as automobile accidents, traumatic life events, physical abuse, and viral infections might generate CFS symptoms. To date, there's still not enough evidence to determine a connection between neuroendocrine abnormalities and specific stressors in CFS.[71]

Sleep abnormalities and sleep disturbances might also lead to CFS symptoms and have been shown to produce an increased production of TNF and IL-6.[72] However, research on the connection between sleep abnormalities, cytokine secretion patterns, and HPA axis alteration hasn't been conducted thus far in patients with CFS. Further probing is required to describe the neuroendocrine features of the syndrome, which calls for studies to identify neuroendocrine activity in larger populations of patients with CFS, including sufferers that fit specific subtypes of the syndrome, test strategies that involve prescription drugs to affect the HPA axis, and evaluation of stress that was previously hypothesized to generate CFS.[73]

Possible human experimental models, which can temporarily recreate the symptoms of CFS to help in identifying biological markers for the ailment, might be brewing sometime in the near future. Long-term research to capture the fluctuations in symptom severity that most CFS patients encounter may assist in bypassing common research obstacles. A CFS symposium series produced by the CFIDS Association of America was designed to analyze the task of the endocrine, immune, circulatory, and neurological systems in CFS. The symposium assembled research collaboration teams and summoned experts to assess findings, shed light on research and funding priorities, and highlighted the most positive next steps for research.[74]

ANALYSIS

When a viral CFS patient coughs, anyone can get infected by breathing in the particles expelled. Several days after the viruses procreate within human bodies, people become sick. Since viruses change and develop over time, CFS patients are advised to get vaccinated yearly. Moreover, caregivers should note that the immune system and autonomic nervous system are two of the primary players in CFS, which focus on the herpesviruses, comprise sensory nerves, and pursue an established model of related disorders such as fibromyalgia.

Part IV

Resolutions

10

NATURAL APPROACHES TO CHRONIC FATIGUE SYNDROME

Chronic fatigue syndrome (CFS) is a medical condition for which there isn't yet a fully refined, conventional drug. Both pharmacological and natural treatments aim at improving the symptoms such as fatigue, anxiety, muscle pains, and depression. Natural treatment, as the name implies, requires acumen for nonchemical intervention for CFS. It's often considered a more "unadulterated" approach that doesn't involve prescription drugs. Ongoing research examines a broad variety of natural treatment methods and introduces new interventions for managing symptoms.[1]

Complementary and alternative medicine (CAM) is the common name used for herbal and homeopathic medicines. These medicines are often administered by a complementary medicine practitioner. Homeopathy is a system of complementary and alternative medicines based on the belief that a distinct disease or syndrome like CFS can be treated by something other than standard medication. Homeopathic remedies are concoctions of substances often so diluted that the main ingredients are barely detectable. Herbal medicines can be administered to patients by drinking a particular plant in powdered or brewed form. Herbal medications use the power of nature to be effective.[2]

SIGNIFICANCE OF APPROACHING CFS NATURALLY: BENEFITS

Discourses are circulating surrounding the different natural approaches to chronic fatigue syndrome. The benefits and drawbacks of addressing CFS naturally are diverse, and the results of experiments and studies fickle. However, a significant number of medical researchers and health advocates favor natural approaches for treating and managing CFS, because these methods can be tested with little or no adverse effects.[3]

Easily Attainable and Less Expensive Treatments

Natural therapies such as herbal and homeopathic remedies are less expensive than chemically processed drugs. Some popular natural herbs such as ginseng, which is known to ward off fatigue, can be bought from the nearest market and can in fact grow at home. Implementing a healthy diet is a natural approach to CFS that compels patients to remove unhealthy and sometimes expensive foods from their diet.[4]

Some oral supplements are easily located at drugstores and in health food stores, as is the case with natural herbs. Supplements are usually less expensive than commercial drugs, since they're widely processed and don't require a prescription. Some methods for improving physical, social, and psychological health, which are proven to be of substantial importance in the treatment of chronic fatigue syndrome, are free: CFS sufferers can exercise and meditate at home.[5]

Less Adverse Effects

Drug dependency is common in CFS patients who take pharmacological medications. Since CFS doesn't have an orthodox prescription, patients tend to self-medicate with over-the-counter (OTC) drugs such as painkillers to reduce discomfort. Erroneous dosage may result in drug abuse or other dire aftershocks. Both OTC and prescription medicines that aren't administered cautiously can cause substance abuse and addiction. Consequently, people suffering from medical conditions sometimes resort to natural approaches, regarding them as safer alternatives to contentious pharmacological drugs.[6]

Natural approaches to CFS are widely used, with or without prescription, as they have fewer adverse side effects than pharmacological drugs. Alternative and supplementary medicines, cognitive behavioral therapy, change in diet, and other natural approaches could easily be subjected to research and clinical trials without diminishing the condition of the patients involved.[7]

Medical Attention to Patients with Allergic Reactions to Drugs

It's not uncommon for CFS clients to be sensitive to some medications such as antidepressants, sedatives, and anticholinergic drugs. The patient instead could ask for supervision and take alternative drugs in order to manage pain and improve symptoms. Individuals with mild CFS can also make use of the recuperative effects of meditation, exercise, and a salubrious diet without the use of any medicinal intervention.[8]

SIGNIFICANCE OF APPROACHING CFS NATURALLY: DRAWBACKS

Although research reports have flooded scientific journals recently, investigators still can't offer a sure answer about the effectiveness of natural approaches in treating CFS. Due to the limited number of randomized controlled trial (RCT) samples, a majority of studies still have the possibility of bias. Some patients respond well to natural approaches but others don't.[9]

Studies have been replicated but the results are typically sparse and inconclusive. The main reasons for bias include inconsistent dosage of an unorthodox medicine, different intervals for physical and psychological therapies, and failure to address the diverse factors of CFS in patients. The studies made on the different interventions have divergent outcomes, thus, further studies and stricter methodologies are encouraged.[10]

Anecdotal Theories

Being termed "natural" doesn't automatically mean that using natural remedies is without risk. People with CFS might self-medicate with natural herbs or homeopathic medicines that they believe would cure their symptoms. However, rigorous studies haven't been conducted. The utility of herbal and homeopathic medicines is primarily based on ancient traditions. Some herbal supplements aren't subjected to research but are still regularly prescribed by alternative medicine practitioners. [11]

Tendency for Self-medication

Patients with chronic fatigue might be swindled by advertisements on the Internet and social media sites about OTC supplements and homeopathic remedies, which allow them to treat themselves without seeking qualified guidance. There's a high risk for side effects of medications in the absence of clinical evidence or at least a few nominal scientific studies. Some advertised medicines are unacknowledged by medical authorities and their manufacturers could be unregulated to a certain extent. [12]

Effects Are Relative to the Patient

Another reason why there's no single, conventional medicine prescribed for CFS is that patients have capricious symptoms and severity levels. The effect of a particular approach can be very beneficial to one patient but tremendously detrimental to the other. For instance, support groups might be able to help CFS patients to cope with their illness through enrichment of social involvement. However, some patients still consider therapy unhelpful and stressful, especially if the support group is comprised of people they're not comfortable with. Drugs sometimes offer the same mixed response. Individual patients have their own level of drug resistance and sensitivity. Thus, they interact with medications differently. [13]

CHANGING THE SOCIAL AND LIVING ENVIRONMENT OF THE PATIENT

The social determinants of a particular medical disorder include the level of education, employment, social status, social support connections, healthy child development, the living environment, and health services available for the patient.[14] These factors can influence the prevalence of a medical disorder in a given population, as well as increase the probability of suffering from a disorder later in life. These factors also help to provide medical researchers and practitioners with a better understanding of how CFS originated and how severely it disturbs the patient. The sufferer's social and living environment can be deeply improved through the implementation of *psychosocial* management techniques.

Improving the Social Environment of the Patient

The CFS patient's social milieu—his home, workplace, and community—proves to be a significant factor affecting his ailment. Only a few studies have sought to ascertain the social determinants of CFS. In one research, it was found out that most CFS patients carry a heavy psychosocial burden.[15] Chronic fatigue sufferers might call themselves "busy people." They often have tedious high-profile or low-paying jobs, as well as unhealthy relationships with other members of society. For example, parents who work outside the home throughout the workday arrive home to cook, care for children, and perform errands for the family. This can be stressful and dreadfully fatiguing by midnight.[16]

People who are very busy with work and frequently put in overtime hours are often stressed due to the expectations they set for themselves. Ignoring rest until they've completed their work, being perfectionists, and setting unrealistic goals may deprive them of sleep and may cause stress and fatigue, which diminishes their energy. Unfortunately, patients with severe cases of CFS are usually those with the fewest health and social support services.[17]

That's because (a) the usual therapies given to medical clients who don't have unyielding CFS have different medication dosage or (b) the method of delivery to those with a less severe form of the syndrome. The results of research on chronic fatigue syndrome are highly variable.

CFS patients with different levels of clinical severity react differently to a particular approach. Repercussions vary from patient to patient, but tweaking the lifestyle of a CFS sufferer in a natural way can jam the symptoms at the very least. Some methods to improve social health in the CFS sufferer are as follows:[18]

- Managing family-related problems;
- Joining a support group;
- Building a healthy relationship with one's doctor; and
- Integrating cognitive behavioral therapy into the patient's lifestyle.

Family Problems

It can become exhausting for people to return to an unhealthy home environment after an interminable day of work. The reasons for this can include altercations with a disloyal spouse or dealing with a problematic teenager, and this can precipitate a CFS patient's depression. Management of patients' relationships with others, especially those who are close to them, such as their own family or relatives, has been shown to minimize the symptoms of CFS. One study found out that patients who have a designated person to care for them, such as a best friend or a spouse, are likely to heal.[19]

Support Groups

Although there are drawbacks to support groups as explained earlier, these groups can also help a person with CFS. The daily activities of a support group can favorably improve CFS patients' conditions. Through the supervision of doctors, a patient becomes active socially, mentally, and physically without overexerting his mental and physical capacities. However, as mentioned, not all patients respond well to support groups.[20]

Some of them are either uncomfortable with the other patients or with their doctors; others prefer isolation. People suffering from a disorder argue that they often can't maintain the physical activity level that's required each day. For example, support groups employ a standard exercise routine based on the physical capacity of its members.

Some may be unable to perform the prescribed activity well, so those patients may be better cured away from others.[21]

Doctor-patient Relationship as a Natural Approach

In one study, 84 percent of 126 children with chronic fatigue syndrome alleged that they felt bullied by authorities such as medical and educational professionals.[22] Eighty-seven percent of them asserted that they lacked support and recognition of their needs. Physicians can help patients meet their sociological and psychological needs through empathic support, which consequently improves patient recovery in a natural manner. A person with CFS won't improve greatly if there's discord between the patient and his doctor. Although it's true that doctors should properly care for their CFS patients, the latter should also believe in their professional caregivers. The two parties should respect one another by communicating in ethical and benevolent ways.[23]

Exercise as a Natural Approach

Generally, inactive patients are considered unhealthy—even those without any diagnosis of disease. Lack of physical activity can be either the cause or effect of CFS, but due to the syndrome, patients tend to exercise less since they become easily fatigued. Exercise is indirectly related to the physiological health of individuals with CFS. As the severity of the condition snowballs, the physical activity of the patient might also decline. Patients who can't participate normally in gym workouts might be left in isolation. Some clients fear post-exertional malaise (PEM), which may lead to setbacks.[24] Therefore, exercising with someone who supports them and matters to them could naturally accelerate healing. There's a vast multitude of research regarding the positive effects of exercise in CFS patients. There are two kinds of physical activities currently examined with effective results for most patients— graded exercise therapy (GET) and pacing.[25]

GET is a form of physical therapy wherein a person exercises at a gentle pace and gradually increases intensity over time. Normally it all starts with simple stretching. The frequency of the activity is increased depending on the CFS patient's ability to cope. In one study, gradual treatment of clients has been shown to produce positive effects. After six months, however, about 30 to 50 percent of the patients who received GET weren't significantly healthier than those who hadn't.[26]

Pacing is another form of physical activity wherein the patient exercises for a certain period of time for as long as he can manage without exacerbating symptoms and triggering post-exertional malaise. Pacing is generally better than graded exercise therapy. About 96 percent of 828 patients who participated in a study in 2008 evaluated pacing as exceedingly helpful.[27]

Psychological Health

People who manage stress using cognitive behavioral therapy (CBT) claim that they effectively reduced symptoms brought on by chronic fatigue syndrome. They also have healthier social lives and respond well to social groups. Cognitive behavioral therapies such as daily meditation and hypnotic therapy could improve the CFS patient's condition. The practice of CBT is effective not only in managing diseases, but also for a better lifestyle.[28]

One study evaluated fifty-three patients who received cognitive behavioral therapy. After treatments, the majority improved their social adjustments (such as exposure to new acquaintances), their outlook on longtime goals, and their fatigue three months later compared to the treatment on the first interval of the study. A six-month follow-up also showed an increase in improvement.[29]

Physical Environment of the CFS Patient

A CFS patient's health is massively influenced by the environment in which he lives. Where the patient resides, where he works, and where he gets treatment also play a seminal role in CFS. It's common advice for people and disease sufferers to live in a place that's comfortable. Clean air and a clean home in an ambient area are weighty considerations when choosing where to live. Although there's been overwhelming research on immunological, nutritional, and sociological factors in the study of CFS, there are relatively few studies on the effects of the environment in which the patient lives and works.[30]

The living environment of an individual could have a mammoth effect on health. For example, in 1990 a study found that poor people living in a neighborhood with wealthy residents are generally healthier than poor people who lived in a neighborhood with poor residents.[31] This is called the "neighborhood effect." The study was based on the mortality rates and incidence of heart disease among the families.[32]

Exposure to Harsh Environments

One study searched for evidence of environmental exposure to CFS.[33] A few patients were found to have environmental and food toxicity before they showed symptoms of CFS. The clients examined had a history of either chemical or food poisoning, such as exposure to pesticides, fish poisoning, sick building syndrome (SBS), Gulf War syndrome (GWS), and many more.[34]

A recent study divulged that exposure to moldy environments such as water-damaged homes or workplaces cause CFS-like illness.[35] It's still unclear whether it's a CFS-related problem or unrelated periphery. The pediatric diagnosis of the illness matched the symptoms of CFS. Further studies on environmental toxicity could provide valuable knowledge about the pathophysiology of chronic fatigue syndrome. Reducing these toxic exposures could act as a natural preventive measure and might also improve the conditions of the individuals suffering from CFS.[36]

NATURAL DRUGS AND SUPPLEMENTS

Natural drugs such as herbal medicines and homeopathic medicines are generally termed safe and effective. Although the majority of these natural remedies do have fewer negative effects, some are not recommended. These alternative drugs usually aren't subjected to research, and most are used in accordance with ancient, traditional practice without proof that they really cure CFS.

Studies have found homeopathy to be effective in CFS. One study found improved reduction in functional limitations and fatigue, and others unearthed symptomatic improvement of CFS.[37]

Ginseng

Ginseng is often marketed to help patients with chronic fatigue syndrome. However, one study found that incorporating ginseng into one's medication had little discernible effect on patients and it failed to show effectively on the Rand vitality index scale.[38]

Mechanism of Action

The hypothesized mechanism of action of complementary medicines describes how the substance is scientifically practical. The benefits of using complementary medications in the treatment of chronic fatigue syndrome are often anecdotal. These experiments are also often judged as biased, so more studies need to be commissioned.[39] Likewise, only trace amounts of the active ingredients are found in alternative medicines. This is often criticized by researchers and doctors, as the dose-response relationship of these medications—which is often incorporated in surveys on therapeutic drugs—can't be gauged. Complementary medicine researchers, however, claim that the more an alternative drug is diluted, the greater it stimulates health. This paradox is still scientifically unexplained.[40]

Side Effects

Homeopathic medicines are diluted in such a way that the main component can be traced in very small amounts. In this way, practitioners argue that side effects and incorrect dosage are prevented. This is often termed as a paradoxical effect similar to placebo but more effective. Homeopathic treatments are considered nontoxic and are made from all-natural herbs and other compounds. The primary drawbacks or adverse effects that a patient feels are symptoms of healing crisis, wherein the CFS patient may feel poor during the initial stages of treatment, but later, as the homeopathic drug is sustained, he gets better.[41]

DIET AND ITS ROLE IN CFS

People who maintain a healthy diet have a better response to diseases including CFS. In terms of natural health, diet—hand in hand with mild exercise—can deeply improve CFS. Compared to homeopathy and other alternative medical treatments, supplements have been far more accepted in the treatment of CFS. Diet management includes drinking supplementary medicines, eating the right food, and pursuing hale habits in order to supply essential nutrients, to enjoy a happier life, and to live a healthier lifestyle. Some scholars postulate that CFS is inflamed by nutritional deficiency, and current research is examining the effects of integrating vitamin and mineral supplements into one's diet.[42]

It's advised that an individual shouldn't skip meals. Multiple smaller meals should be eaten daily and include nutritious foods from all the food groups, which not only maintains a balanced diet, but also regulates the CFS patient's blood glucose at a healthy level. This also inhibits excess insulin production and regulates cortisol levels, which then helps to maintain a healthy weight and appetite.[43]

Processed foods may contain high levels of sodium and sugar, which tends to increase the body's insulin level. That in turn makes the person feel hungry and increases the cortisol levels in the person's blood. Whole grains such as cereals, oat cookies, or multigrain biscuits better balance insulin levels and control the level of glucose in blood. These types of foods are better choices when considering daily snacks rather than those high in salt, calories, and sugar.[44]

Supplements are regarded as far safer than herbal medicines. They are for the prevention and treatment of chronic fatigue syndrome, because researchers have hypothesized that CFS is also set off by an imbalance of nutrients. Essential body nutrients may not be successfully incorporated into a patient's diet, thus a doctor may prescribe supplements to normalize this imbalance.[45]

By extension, some medical disorders such as CFS also deplete important vitamins and minerals, as well as drain *phytochemicals* from the organs. Ingestion of vitamins and supplements would also be strategic, especially when combined with proper diet. Dietary change is a key to being healthy. Not only does it require dedication, but it also helps one to live healthfully using a natural approach.[46]

L-carnitine

L-carnitine is an amino acid that's vital to cell, brain, heart, and muscular function by infusing the human organism with energy. It prevents fatty acids from accumulating in the *mitochondria*, which helps in the metabolism of energy. It occurs naturally in the body. However, some people have naturally low levels of L-carnitine. Because of its significance to the CFS sufferer's metabolism, low levels of L-carnitine in the organs may lead to symptoms such as general fatigue, physical weakness, and muscular pain. Those suffering from insufficiency are thus required to have L-carnitine supplementation.[47]

Evidence has been found that patients with CFS also have L-carnitine deficiency, but research results are mixed.[48] A third of the samples in one trial responded well to L-carnitine supplements, drastically improving their well-being, even when they previously had been severely affected by CFS. The other two-thirds, however, didn't respond positively.[49]

New reviews, however, prove the effectiveness of L-carnitine in CFS patients. A systematic assessment of two studies in 2006 found that L-carnitine improved the overall health of patients, although there was no placebo control.[50] L-carnitine is vital and has been often used as a supplement for a variety of heart conditions such as diabetes, heart attack, rheumatic heart disease, and more. It's also used as supplementary medicine for thyroid disease and even for AIDS medications.

Magnesium

Patients with CFS are more likely to suffer magnesium deficiency as well. Stress hormones, which increase in those who suffer from CFS, slash the magnesium levels of the red blood cells in the body.[51] The many studies conducted on the effects of magnesium in the patient have had mixed results. Some studies reported favorable effects but were unable to provide rock-solid conclusions. A recent review in 2008 asserted that magnesium supplements still can't be deemed an official treatment for chronic fatigue syndrome.[52]

Essential Fatty Acids

Patients with CFS are also found to have low essential fatty acid levels. It is postulated that the low levels of essential fatty acids (EFA) caused CFS symptoms and other dysfunctions in the immune, endocrine, and sympathetic nervous systems. One study examined the effect of EFA intervention on post-viral fatigue by using evening primrose oil and fish oil. The patients showed significant improvement in their symptoms such as fatigue and depression.[53]

Researchers tried to replicate the study for chronic fatigue syndrome, using sunflower oil as their medium rather than paraffin, as in the first study. Research, however, arrived at a different outcome. A possible explanation can be deduced from the difference of symptomatic criteria and the medium used to supply EFAs.[54]

Positive effects were shown in another study, where almost thirty patients who were ill for about six years were subjected to trial. They were given EFA supplements along with cognitive behavioral therapy and graded exercise therapy. After three months, the condition of twenty-seven patients improved.[55]

Vitamin B12

Vitamin B12, or cobalamin, is vital for DNA synthesis and normal functioning of the brain and the nervous system. It helps the tissues to tender more red blood cells. A deficiency in vitamin B12 makes an individual lethargic and leads to the development of anemia. Although fatigue and depression are typical symptoms of CFS and vitamin B12 deficiency, there's little scientific data to prove that they're directly related. Like most research, one way to find out is to examine whether incorporating vitamin B12 supplements could help CFS.[56]

Studies over the years have shown that vitamin B12 supplements offer therapeutic and pharmacological effects for CFS. A total of four studies examined vitamin B12 effects on patients suffering with chronic fatigue syndrome. Three of the studies exhibited desirable results.[57] It was concluded that as the dosage is increased above the amount needed to correct vitamin B12 deficiency, the effectiveness also increases. Fifty to 80 percent of the patients experienced less fatigue and improved stamina. In the fourth study, however, vitamin B12 was administered at very low doses and didn't prove effective. [58]

Evidence was found that 40 to 100 percent of CFS patients have eccentric red blood cells called *nondiscocytes*. [59] It was postulated that these abnormal erythrocytes impair proper cellular respiration and oxidation in the CFS patient's body. In an open trial, vitamin B12 was administered to CFS patients. Half responded well, evincing enhanced well-being within twenty-four hours. Researchers observed decreased deformation and a significant reduction of the nondiscocytes in their blood. However, the remaining participants weren't affected at all and the structure of their red blood cells never transmuted. [60]

It was settled in the study that supplementation with vitamin B12 lessens fatigue, reduces physical pain, and also improves blood circulation, thus signifying vitamin B12 as a future treatment for CFS. However, an experiment in 2010 revealed that incorporating vitamin B12 into patients' diets didn't have any significant effects on fatigue or other CFS symptoms. [61] The contrasting outcomes suggest the need for further research.

Candida albicans

Candida albicans are the microorganisms that cause yeast infection and *thrush*. They normally thrive in the large intestines, genitals, mouth, and even on the skin. *Candida* overgrown has been suggested as one cause of CFS. People who suffer from candidiasis are known to exhibit symptoms of CFS. One clinical study identified *candida albicans* as a causal agent of CFS by triggering immune dysfunction caused by yeast overgrowth. [62]

The study also showed a beneficial effect of the *candida* diet on a significant number of patients. Many health experts and CFS patients practiced supervised, independent *candida* diets. In response, a new study placed CFS patients on either a low-sugar, low-yeast diet (LSLY) or healthy eating (HE) program. It was found out that the two interventions were not as efficacious in terms of fatigue levels. One bias could be that the LSLY diet was too complicated and not practical. [63]

Balanced Nutrition

Nutritional balancing is extremely gentle and safe, which can't be said of other treatments used today. Vegetarianism, fasting, and other extreme diets worsen the problems in many instances.[64] A specific three-step program in eliminating fatigue through natural approaches is advisable. First, a patient should incorporate pacing. Second, an individual with CFS is instructed to take cognitive behavioral therapy. Lastly, one should also eat nutritious foods.[65] Experts often advise others to eat about five times a day but in small amounts. Low-carbohydrate, high-protein foods are recommended in the morning and in between meals to help stabilize blood sugar and to replenish energy.

According to studies, mornings are the best part of the day to consume food.[66] Upon waking up, blood glucose levels decline and cortisol levels rise. Eating in the morning balances blood sugar and reduces cortisol levels in the blood. Balanced blood glucose replenishes energy, and the reduction in cortisol leads to a lower appetite. Moreover, the levels of cortisol and blood sugar are retained throughout the day, thus making an individual energized and satiated.[67]

According to scientists, in order to suppress fatigue, one should begin by replenishing the body by eating the right foods.[68] The consumption of fresh fruits, uncooked vegetables, nuts, and freshly milled cereals are recommended. Drinking supplements alone is highly unadvisable. Supplements or alternative medications cannot take the place of well-balanced nutrition. Before taking a supplement or alternative medicine, one should discuss it with a well-qualified health professional first.

SLEEP IS A NATURAL APPROACH

It's sensible to strictly observe bedtimes in order to set one's body clock properly. Should there be changes in sleeping patterns, it's recommended that healthcare professionals be involved with the monitoring. Patients may experience sleep disturbances like insomnia and sleep-wake reversals.[69]

Lack of sleep would then distress an individual's mood and energy level, which are essential for cognitive and other physical functions.

Sleep can determine a CFS patient's performance level at work. "Recharging" sleep helps to prevent or lessen the person's feelings of exhaustion, or worse, fatigue. Patients must remain conscientious with their sleep schedules.[70]

ANALYSIS

Although the pathophysiology of CFS remains a mystery, different treatment trials have been advanced to improve the patient's symptoms. Many researchers and sufferers unceasingly seek ways to cure CFS and its symptoms in a manner that makes the patients feel safe and comfortable. When considering safe methods of tackling CFS, natural approaches immediately come to mind.

11

PHARMACOLOGICAL APPROACHES TO CHRONIC FATIGUE SYNDROME

The pharmacological management of chronic fatigue syndrome (CFS) is geared toward alleviating the most debilitating and disruptive symptoms of the disorder as prioritized by the client. This view is also shared by the Centers for Disease Control, since each individual experiences varying manifestations, degrees of severity, and responses to medication. The term "management" is an appropriate term to use because there's no single drug or line of prescription medication that can completely cure the complex nature of CFS. Rather, a highly individualized approach is more effective, since one drug may work for one client but not for another.[1]

Frequently used medications to relieve symptoms can range from over-the-counter products to some controlled substances, for which the cost and availability differs, too. The efficacy of these medications is on a case-by-case basis, so it's best to consult with a physician and a reliable healthcare team. Clients must always keep in mind that managing this disorder by using prescribed medications is only effective when taken as instructed by a physician. This includes the timely consumption of the drug and taking it only for the specific length of time prescribed by a physician in order to maximize the benefits, prevent long-term adverse reactions, and avoid drug-to-drug interactions that can further harm the individual. Hence, cooperation between the client and the health team provides the best chance for successful CFS management.[2]

ANTIPYRETICS, ANALGESICS, AND ANTI-INFLAMMATORY MEDICATIONS

Chronic fatigue syndrome was once called the "yuppie flu," with the flulike symptoms including fever and muscular pain among apparent CFS sufferers. Antipyretics for fever, analgesics for pain, and anti-inflammatories for inflammation were commonly prescribed at the time. Medications that can relieve these symptoms include nonsteroidal anti-inflammatory drugs (NSAIDs) such as ibuprofen, aspirin, naprosensodium, and feldene.[3]

Indications and Mechanisms of Action

Inhibition of the prostaglandin synthesis, mainly of the *cyclooxygenase* 2 type of prostaglandin responsible for smooth muscle contraction and relaxation results in reduced fever, pain, and inflammation—all symptoms of which CFS patients complain. These should be taken an hour before or two hours after a meal, but if adverse reactions follow, the drugs may be taken with milk.[4]

Benefits, Drawbacks, and Side Effects

NSAIDs are prescribed because they work with the same potency as—but without the ravaging side effects of—steroids or narcotics. Adverse effects include tinnitus or ringing in the ear, *pharyngitis*, prolonged bleeding time, hepatitis, and increased potassium (also known as hyperkalemia). Chronic fatigue syndrome sufferers are also advised not to take alcohol and to avoid hazardous activities while on medication. It's also important to talk to the physician when combining drugs in this class to avert kidney damage and gastrointestinal bleeding, especially when using the drug on a long-term basis. It's important to schedule an appointment for kidney and liver function tests regularly, so that health care providers can monitor the dose or to refashion the prescription.[5]

ANTIDEPRESSANTS

Mild doses of antidepressants are prescribed to clients with CFS because they help manage mood swings and are believed to improve the quality of sleep and sometimes decrease pain. There are however, different types of antidepressants and their use is controversial. Selective serotonin reuptake inhibitors, or SSRIs, and selective norepinephrine reuptake inhibitors, or SNRIs, include fluoxetine, sertraline, paroxetine, venlafaxine, trazodone, and bupropion. Another type commonly used is the tricyclic antidepressant, or TCA, named for its molecular structure containing three atom rings. Examples of TCA include doxepin, amitriptyline, desipramine, and nortriptyline.[6]

Patients diagnosed with CFS tend to respond promisingly to lower doses of antidepressant drugs than the average doses typically used for depression in patients without the syndrome. In some cases, CFS sufferers can't tolerate the usual doses used for patients without CFS. Since it may take several weeks before the drugs have the desired effect, it's best to work with closely with a professional caregiver regarding pharmacologic therapy for depression.[7]

Indications and Mechanisms of Action

SSRI, SNRI, and TCA act on neurotransmitters such as serotonin and norepinephrine. These neurotransmitters, which are comparatively lower in CFS clients, are responsible for sleep and wake cycles and for bursts of energy. Only the smallest doses of these drugs are prescribed in order to prevent addiction and dependency.[8]

Benefits, Drawbacks, and Side Effects

Depression is believed not to originate from the disorder itself, but as a by-product of the continual fatigue that hinders the individual from participating in the normal social activities that one is accustomed to do. The use of SSRI, SNRI, and TCA is applicable but may take several weeks to enrich mood. The important thing is to remind the client to continue taking the medication as prescribed even when the desired effects aren't yet felt. However, there's an arsenal of side effects from antidepressant drugs, such as the following:[9]

- Drowsiness;
- Constipation;
- Hyperglycemia;
- Dry mouth;
- Orthostatic hypotension;
- Palpitations;
- Blurred vision;
- Urine retention;
- Rashes;
- Weight gain;
- Abdominal pain;
- Increased salivation;
- Decreased immune function;
- Decreased sexual desire; and
- Congestive heart failure.

These reactions need to be taken into serious consideration, and a complete clinical history must be completed before these drugs are prescribed in order to avoid contraindications for other past or present conditions. There are also specific instructions to be taken to heart, for instance, abstaining from all forms of alcoholic beverages, avoiding excessive sun exposure, and discontinuing the use of certain herbs that affect the potency of antidepressants such as St. John's wort and evening primrose. Consultation with a doctor is vital, as these medications must be taken at specific times during the day to maintain the drug blood level, and they can't be discontinued abruptly, as this can lead to bewildering thoughts, contemplation of suicide, or psychosis. [10]

ANXIOLYTICS

Some CFS clients may report anxiety or panic attacks. However, the value of anti-anxiety medications is questionable and they must be used only when the alms outweigh the adverse effects. Benzodiazepines, a class of anxiolytic commonly used, include alprazolam, diazepam, lorazepam, midazolam hydrochloride, and oxazepam. [11]

Indications and Mechanism of Action

The specific action of benzodiazepines is unknown, but it's believed to affect a neurotransmitter called *gamma-aminobutyric acid* or GABA, which is responsible for the excitability of the central nervous system (CNS). Benzodiazepines are also known to depress the CNS at the brain level.[12]

Benefits, Drawbacks, and Side Effects

The efficacy of benzodiazepines is based on both the client's responsiveness to the drug and his commitment to adhere to the treatment plan. It's also important to inform prescribers about all the medications one is currently taking to avoid drug-to-drug interactions. Anxiolytics are available in different forms, such as oral gels, injectable solutions, and tablets, so it's important that the CFS patient asks the physician about the best option for his condition. Side effects are closely similar to those of an antidepressant but they can also vary among individuals. Drowsiness, hypotension, visual disturbances, abdominal discomfort, nausea, and hepatic dysfunction can occur. Chronic fatigue sufferers with sensitivity to soy protein should avoid soy, since it can affect liver function tests.[13]

SLEEPING PILLS

Insomnia is one of the most reported symptoms of CFS and probably the most debilitating, since lack of sleep aggravates the client's fatigue. Some of the popular sleeping pills prescribed are sedative hypnotics like zolpidem tartrate, eszopiclone, orphenadrine, melatonin, and zopiclone. These are usually given in low doses to provide a peaceful and restful sleep. When larger doses are necessary, they are used with meticulous care.[14]

Indications and Mechanisms of Action

Sleeping pills are a combination of different classes of drugs ranging from antihistamines, antidepressants, or sedative-hypnotics. The main mechanism of action is to decrease the ability of neurons to fire signals and excite neighboring neurons located within the *limbic system* and the CNS, thereby allowing for a restful sleep. However, sleeping pills may also be required, as well. Antihistamines are mainly respiratory tract drugs used to treat certain allergies, but the side effects include sedation. Therefore, these drugs are also used to manage insomnia, especially for newly diagnosed clients, while antidepressants reportedly improve sleep patterns.[15]

Benefits, Drawbacks, and Side Effects

Sedatives are effective to help curb sleep deprivation when used correctly. Sedatives are beneficial, but like any medication, the CFS sufferer must be evaluated first to determine what drug is appropriate and how long it should be used. The adverse effects of sleeping pills are the same as for antidepressants: hallucinations, vertigo, peripheral edema, ear discomfort, conjunctivitis, bronchitis, and fever. Ironically, too many sedatives can lead to insomnia. Adverse reactions are mostly dose related, so a dose reduction might be merited if the reactions become too bothersome for the clients. It's essential to check with a sleep specialist because nonrestorative sleep may be present even while taking the medications. A careful sleep study should be urged if that happens.[16]

ANTIVIRALS

Antivirals such as acyclovir, valacyclovir, and valganciclovir are commonly used for CFS, since it is thought that viral infection may be one cause of the disorder. This relates to several reported cases of Epstein-Barr virus, herpesviruses, and human cytomegalovirus (HCMV) in CFS clients and the success of antivirals in significantly reducing overall fatigue.[17]

Indications and Mechanisms of Actions

The mechanism of action of antiviral drugs differs depending on their subclasses, yet the goal remains to prohibit the virus from reproducing by attacking the viral DNA chain. This can be achieved by attacking the virus's nucleus, thus preventing synthesis. Clients are advised to take these drugs on an empty stomach or to consume them with liquids such as skim milk, juice, coffee, or tea. It should also be noted that eating a high-calorie, high-fat meal might hinder the absorption process of the gut.[18]

Benefits, Drawbacks, and Side Effects

Studies confirm the effects of using antiviral medications to improve CFS. However, this may not be true for all CFS clients. The use of these drugs is largely dependent upon the symptoms and client's response to the treatment. Antivirals should be used cautiously because inappropriate use can lead to overdose and resistant viruses. Adverse reactions may include the following:[19]

- Agitation;
- Amnesia;
- Confusion;
- Hallucinations;
- Bronchitis;
- Lung edema;
- Muscle pain;
- Anorexia;
- Diarrhea;
- Nausea and vomiting;
- Kidney stones;
- Hematuria; and
- *Stevens-Johnson syndrome.*

Abdominal pain must be reported immediately to the prescriber because this may mean gastro-intestinal bleeding. Clients must also note that drug-to-drug interactions may influence efficacy of medications. For instance, using antidepressants and antivirals together can cause respiratory depression, thus they cannot be taken simultaneously. Chronic fatigue syndrome patients who are also on oral contraceptives must be warned about their decreased effectiveness when other medicines are being taken, and an alternate method of contraception should be used.[20]

ANTIBIOTICS

Some clients report chronic fatigue soon after being infected with a respiratory disorder called mononucleosis, which is treated with antibiotics. However, antibiotics are composed of a wide array of medications, so a single class or a combination from distinct classes can be prescribed based on the client's medical history. Some of the antibiotic groups commonly used are aminoglycosides, gentamycin, streptomycin sulfate, and neomycin. Penicillins that also work include the following:[21]

- Ampicillin;
- Amoxicillin;
- Cloxacillin;
- Oxacillin; and
- Penicillin G.

Other effective medications are as follows:

- Cefaclor;
- Cefixime;
- Ceftazadine;
- Ceftriaxone;
- Cephalexin;
- Doxycyline;
- Tetracycline;
- Hydrochloride;
- Ciprofloxacin;
- Levofloxacin;
- Norfloxacin; and
- Sparfloxacin.

Indications and Mechanisms of Action

Antibiotics act by killing bacteria. Cell wall manufacture is prevented during bacterial multiplication. Most antibiotics are taken as a five- to seven-day continuous treatment, as clients are advised to take the drug at specific times, every twelve or eight hours, to stabilize the drug blood level. This makes the drug more effective in combating the bacteria that's causing infection. Antibiotic administration is more effective when a bacteria culture and sensitivity test identifies the specific microorganism causing the problem. Although this may take time, the first dose can be given while awaiting test results.[22]

Benefits, Drawbacks, and Side Effects

Like antiviral medications, antibiotics should be taken cautiously because unsupervised use results in resistant bacteria, a more serious medical condition to treat. If taken correctly, the rate of effectiveness is high and symptoms of the infection usually abate after three days. Patients must be warned to take the drug for the entire course of treatment for complete healing. Adverse effects, such as oral lesion, *enterocolitis*, nephropathy, and *agranulocytosis* must be reported to the physician. Moreover, hypersensitivity reactions are common, thus testing and asking about any allergies before dispensation is essential.[23]

ANTIPROTOZOALS

A protozoal infection such as pneumocystis carinii pneumonia (PCP) isn't very common, occurring only when one's immune system is severely compromised. This is undeniably true among CFS clients, so the use of antiprotozoal medications could be compulsory. These drugs include atovaquone and pentamidine.[24]

Indications and Mechanisms of Action

Antiprotozoals must be used carefully in patients with impaired liver and kidney function as they may further damage said organs. Patients should take the medication with food, which enhances absorption. The exact mechanism of action of antiprotozoals is unknown, but it's believed that they interfere with the reproduction of susceptible organisms by blocking the DNA and RNA. Drugs must be used with extreme caution in clients with preexisting disorders such as hypertension, hypotension, hypoglycemia, hypocalcemia, diabetes, and pancreatitis.[25]

Benefits, Drawbacks, and Side Effects

The whole point of antimicrobials such as antiprotozoals is to treat the principal cause of infection that may be the cradle for CFS. Thus clients need to be monitored closely during therapy due to the high risk of concurrent respiratory infection. This is a concern that needs to be addressed immediately by the doctor and the entire health care team.[26]

Adverse effects include vertigo, headache, dizziness, seizures, darkened urine, increased urination, metallic taste in the mouth, vaginal candidiasis, joint pains, and rashes. This drug can also escalate liver enzymes and lessen sodium and glucose levels, so CFS clients with preexisting conditions upsetting these blood serums must be monitored closely. Antiprotozoals are also protein bound, so they must be used thoughtfully with other protein-bound medications and checked for toxicity when combined.[27]

NEW ADVANCES IN PHARMACOLOGICAL TREATMENT

Vagus nerve stimulation, antivirals to attack pathogens, glial cell inhibitors to cease immune activations, and surgical adjustment of the vagus nerve are possible treatments of the future. A drug called Ibudilast was used in Japan to inhibit glial cell activation by discouraging the production of proflammatory cytokine, and its blood vessel–dilating and neuron-protecting effects prove beneficial in the treatment of stroke and asthma.[28]

Ibudilast is also appropriate for nerve pain because it regulates glial cell activation and is capable of stopping replication of viruses. The National Institutes of Health have been funding experiments in the United States to determine the drug's effectiveness in treating addiction so that it could be used in the future for CFS patients suffering from substance addiction. Since herpesviruses residing in the sensory nerve complexes might be shielded from antiviral drugs and antibodies, it may be easier to stop glial cell activation. Moreover, other types of viruses might be causing the malady.[29]

Rintatolimod

Rintatolimod is a new drug that's designed to target viruses at the molecular level. Rintatolimod contains nucleic acid components believed to serve two purposes at the same time: it acts as an immune system inducer and an antiviral. However, in 2009, the FDA rejected rintatolimod as a treatment of CFS and vetoed its sale in U.S. markets, asserting that it wasn't proven be to be safe or effective. At present, the pharmaceutical company developing the drug is still performing tests and analyses on rintatolimod in order to gain approval.[30]

Interferons

Interferons, or IFNs, belong to a class of glycoproteins responsible for antiviral activity. These proteins inhibit virus production by propagating white blood cells (called leucocytes and fibroblasts), which engulf invading pathogens. There are two types: type I (alpha and beta interferon) and type II (gamma interferon), the former being more of an antiviral component than the latter. Type II is voided by CD8 T cells and the helper T subset of CD4 cells that are used to stimulate various antigens. It's also distinctively different because it's used to patch up chronic *granulomatous disease*.[31]

Cortisones

Evidence indicates that the reactivity of the HPA axis decreases in adult CFS patients when compared with control subjects. Hydrocortisone treatment produced minimum development, whereas oral administration of low doses of hydrocortisone showed improvement in the clinical condition of about 30 percent of a select group of CFS patients.[32] An oral hydrocortisone deployed in other research also shows some improvement when measured through fluctuations in wellness scores. Still, there weren't any substantial changes in fatigue and activity in this study. The search for a specific cause in regard to the generalized symptomology of CFS doesn't seem to be the most appropriate approach to use.

Immunotherapy

The immune system is thought to be one of the culprits for acquiring CFS, so physicians and patients are looking into the possibility of boosting the immune system to improve symptoms. Immunoglobulins are a group of plasma proteins that help protect the body by fighting infection. Immunoglobulin G, or IgG, is the primary immunoglobulin in human serum. It can move through the placental barrier, thereby allowing the mother to pass on immunity to the fetus before birth. Immunoglobulin G is the major antibody for viruses, bacteria, and toxins. The efficacy among CFS sufferers is still individualized; therefore more research needs to be done before the administration of immunoglobulins.[33]

Rituximab is an antineoplastic drug that's used to treat Hodgkin's lymphoma, a form of blood cancer. The direct correlation between CFS and rituximab isn't well established but clinical trials have been done, with some clients reported improvement after taking rituximab. However, the drug is still open for trials to further develop the ultimate remedial plan (curing CFS completely) and to prove its efficacy for CFS. Patients on this medication are encouraged to avoid tyramine-rich foods and drinks such as smoked meats, wine, cheese, coffee, bananas, cola, and tea, because these may cause further tumors. Likewise, the use of antineoplastic agents for patients without cancer is controversial because the drug can also injure healthy cells, which may further aggravate the client's condition. Clients on rituximab are susceptible to irregular heart rhythms and fatal low blood pressure, hence strict cardiac monitoring is essential.[34]

Hormones

Other drug classes for CFS hormonal therapy include steroid, cortisol, and thyroid hormone replacement. Clinical trials continue to prove the success of these medications in treating CFS. Although some CFS clients may find relief with these drugs, it's best to consult a doctor before taking hormones to avoid dangerous side effects. Long-term effects of hormonal medications such as steroids can result in heart failure, seizures, blood clots, inflammation of the pancreas, susceptibility to infections, acute adrenal insufficiency, and a *cushingoid* state of the body due to toxicity. Hormones must be used carefully, especially in conjunction with other medications, to prevent adverse reactions due to drug interaction.[35]

IMPORTANCE OF TAKING ALL POTENTIAL SIDE EFFECTS SERIOUSLY

The dangers of side effects from medications are real and should be taken to heart. Medications that enter the CFS patient's body are digested in the stomach, metabolized and synthesized by the liver metabolites and other drug particles, and filtered by the kidneys. These organs are affected when medications aren't used correctly or when used for prolonged periods without the oversight of a physician. There's also a risk of severe, life-threatening allergies, so it's wise not to take side effects lightly. The following paragraphs explain medication side effects that pose a great danger to overall health.

Systemic Anaphylaxis

Among the major effects of drugs are mild to severe allergies. Mild allergies may present minor symptoms such as rashes and itchy skin. Severe allergic reactions, however, can lead to anaphylaxis and anaphylactic shock. Responses include hives, wheezing, flushing, nausea and vomiting, *dyspnea*, increased mucus production, and feelings of generalized anxiety. The respiratory, cardiovascular and gastrointestinal systems are greatly affected. The most dangerous symptoms are wheezing and dyspnea, which indicates that the airway is swelling. If air passage is blocked for a while, it can result to death.[36]

The aim of anaphylaxis management is prevention. Before a drug is prescribed, clients are asked about any allergies such as egg, fish, specific drugs, or contrast media. Patients are taught which symptoms to watch out for, as well as those that need to be managed immediately, like dyspnea and wheezing. However, prevention isn't a foolproof plan when it comes to drug allergies because some clients may be allergic to a medication without exhibiting symptoms the first time it was administered.[37]

Increased Cholesterol, Fatty Liver, and Liver Damage

The liver is a processer of nutrients and medications. This organ works diligently to ensure that drugs are metabolized in a way that delivers them to the parts of the body where they are needed. Most drugs can cause increases in cholesterol, leading to fatty liver, which can progress to liver damage. The best treatment is of course prevention; CFS clients must have their liver function tested and cholesterol levels checked regularly, especially when taking drugs for prolonged periods of time. It's essential to help the liver manage lipids and cholesterol by practicing a balanced, low-fat diet.[38]

Kidney Failure

Kidney failure is a tricky side effect of the medications that may be offered to CFS sufferers. The kidney, responsible for sifting out waste products including excessive drug residues, is a steadfast organ. The problem is that a person won't experience major symptoms of kidney failure until the kidneys fail. The kidneys try to compensate for loss of function over time until they can no longer cope. Clients with CFS should be warned about the prolonged usage of pain relievers such as NSAIDs because this is the usual cause of kidney damage. Medications, especially NSAIDs, shouldn't be abused. Clients should have their *creatinine* and blood urea nitrogen (BUN) routinely checked for signs of kidney damage in order to halt its progression.[39]

If kidney damage isn't managed, it can lead to end-stage kidney failure, or ESRD, wherein dialysis is required, which is expensive and has many complications. Other options include kidney transplantation, but the waiting list is long and it can take years to find a suitable kidney. People with CFS should be monitored to preserve their kidney function while still possible.[40]

Many substances have been used in an attempt to cure CFS. Antivirals, anticholinergics, hormones, nicotinamide adenine dinucleotide (NAD), and antidepressants have been tried without conclusive, positive results thus far. On the flip side, steroid treatments show evidence of decreased fatigue.[41] Low doses of nortriptylin at bedtime suggest improved sleep and diminished pain in the patient. For musculoskeletal complaints, nonsteroidal anti-inflammatory agents and acetaminophen might be effective.[42] Also, reports indicate that fibromyalgia, introduced earlier in this book, is improved using antidepressant medications.[43]

ANALYSIS

Pharmacological CFS medications should be used in moderation. Too much of anything, when taken incorrectly, does more harm than good—no matter how good it makes a person feel or how much it improves one's symptoms. It's vital that physicians oversee the prescription of medications and that patients follow their instructions exactly. CFS patients must report any new symptoms or side effects that they experience to their doctors. The treatment plan for CFS is individualized for every sufferer, and pharmacological approaches may not work depending on the individual and other factors. Therefore, individuals with CFS should take medications with extra caution and "listen to their body."[44]

12

ADDRESSING THE MIND

It's inevitable that chronic fatigue syndrome (CFS) patients undergo mental and psychological issues brought about by the syndrome. The following chapter focuses on how to deal with psychological matters that weren't already covered in chapter 9, as well as how to deal with CFS-related stress in the comfort of one's home.

MENTAL ISSUES

How Chronic Fatigue Syndrome Affects Memory

CFS is shown to be associated with deficits in verbal and nonverbal memory tasks.[1] Patients may find it tiring to recall things that require rapid cognition of short-term or working memory. Fatigue brought on by CFS affects the retrospective memory of patients. Retrospective memory includes the memory of what's known: the informational content, such as people of acquaintance, events that happened previously, and other existing information that folks have about themselves and others.[2]

However, fatigue doesn't affect *prospective* memory—remembering *when* to act.[3] This is a pattern of memory that involves "remembering to do planned or intended actions" or activities at an appropriate time.[4] Retrospective memory is important in order for the CFS patient to function effectively in everyday life. It even encompasses daily, routine activities. Patients would then need a daily plan of activities and to remember to cross out what's already been done. However, to avoid overwhelming the patient with his tasks, a long list isn't effective.

In order to avoid creating anxiety and agitation in the patient, the list should break down the tasks, for example, by listing only the first three priorities. After that, patients can reward themselves with some rest or a small incentive for finishing the tasks as a kind of mini-celebration. This activity employs the method of pacing—tackling tasks in increments of time or effort. Pacing is a strategy that encourages CFS patients to find a balance between rest and activity and to live with the physical limitations imposed by CFS. Pacing also helps the patients avoid the detrimental effects of deconditioning, should they fall into drawn-out periods of inactivity.

Self-efficacy and CFS

Psychological factors are found to predict health outcomes—a person's feelings of self-efficacy were associated with CFS.[5] Self-efficacy is defined as the extent or strength of an individual's belief in his own ability to complete tasks and reach goals.[6] Fatigue, depression, and overall self-efficacy are undeniably related to cognitive failures. People with CFS tend to be more depressed than those with many other illnesses. In effect, the lack of motivation associated with depression may lead to low self-efficacy, which in turn leads to cognitive failures.[7] People should not minimize, or much worse, overlook chronic fatigue syndrome. Patients can't treat the mind without treating the health of the whole body and vice versa. People with this disorder have to press on with motivation and perseverance.

Financial Pressures Related to Chronic Fatigue Syndrome

CFS pervasively affects many areas of the patient's life and may even cause financial hardship. The majority of families with little ones face increased expenditures, indicating that some families might experience financial problems caused by caring for a child while also suffering from CFS.[8] Higher expenditures can result in more debt, which only increases the guilt that CFS patients experience when their illness prevents them from working.[9]

STAYING HAPPY AS A CFS PATIENT

It is difficult to believe in one's own ability to prevent or relieve illness—more so when one faces a chronic, seemingly irrepressible illness.[10] However, the mind is powerful, so if patients with CFS can't stop themselves from feeling fatigued, their only recourse is to turn their minds toward positivity and optimism. Thus, CFS patients must accept every new day as a challenge.

Coping Strategies and Their Effects

Individuals with CFS often have to rework their coping mechanisms in order to deal with this disabling chronic syndrome. Cognitive functioning deficits may impair the patient's ability to employ a wide variety of coping strategies, and changing those strategies could refresh the mind again and again.[11] Pursuing viable ways to recover from the syndrome requires creativity and drive.

Optimism

Some people with CFS view the disorder as uncontrollable, which may lead to pessimism and emotion-focused coping. In turn, these coping styles and pessimistic attitudes may lead to poorer health outcomes.[12] CFS inevitably affects emotional well-being. Research suggests that maintaining social activities and a sense of optimism correspond to more positive mental composite scores. This means that the more a patient feels destitute, the more he's drawn to poor outcomes.

Maintaining activities and remaining positive both appear to be related to heightened functionality.[13] Day by day, CFS patients need to "maintain altitude" of their emotions, energy levels, patience, acceptance, and understanding of their condition. Each new day necessitates a positive mind-set among patients with CFS, and the people around them must try fiercely to understand and get along with them, because no one's to blame. No one chooses such an illness. Coping with CFS is about making joy more contagious than it already is.

Acceptance

Embracing the mind means accepting oneself, physically linking oneself to the biological chemicals one is born with, and accepting one's effects on human behavior. This is connected to how recovery or alleviation of symptoms may hinge on the sufferers' perception that they're in control of their syndrome. Psychosocial disturbances are of course linked to one's happiness, despite being a CFS patient.[14]

The key is acceptance, as well as happiness, when managing CFS, and this requires effort from the patient and the people around him. Accepting the disorder is a major step in dealing with CFS in a more effective manner. Since the malady exists, the patient is best served by focusing on solutions rather than negative emotions like sadness or depression, which can lead to immobility.[15]

Acceptance is a great challenge the patient and the people around him must face bravely. Surely no one would ever want to have CFS; however, having CFS is not a choice nor is it within one's control. Friends may recommend health professionals who can take care of him.[16]

Social Disengagement or Isolation

Some people who suffer from CFS isolate themselves because of physical limitations: perhaps in order to preserve their energy, or on the negative side, perhaps they feel inadequate. Other patients eliminate socialization and time spent with their friends because of very low energy levels. CFS sufferers likely prefer staying home and resting rather than attending parties.[17]

By disengaging themselves from the people in their lives, patients conceivably risk losing them in the long run. Humans are social beings—it's only natural to mingle with others outside the immediate family. It's also the right of every child to play and be happy. As people get older and mature further, play becomes different and they reestablish themselves in a more complex manner. Patients with CFS must continue interacting with others rather than staying at home, which may even result in oversleeping and overeating. CFS is always a balance between managing time and energy. Chronic fatigue syndrome sufferers could enjoy some "alone time" while ambling in the park with a pet.[18]

Patients could also maximize family interaction without overexerting themselves simply by watching their children play at the park; if the patient feels like dozing off, he could place a mat on the grass and sleep there. At safe levels, sunlight is actually a great source of energy. If a patient is too tired to function at the office, a fifteen-minute nap should help, whereupon the sufferer can resume work again. Surely all employees know that an eight-hour job isn't really a cakewalk, because everyone, even a nation's president, needs time to relax.[19]

Among CFS patients, behavioral disengagement is related to worsening mental composite scores.[20] Social disengagement is clearly a maladaptive coping style for people with CFS. Much like the rest and proper nutrition required to get through the day, CFS patients also need motivation to stay positive while living with CFS. As everyone knows, it's not as easy as simply reading motivational quotes, but with effort, people can ditch chronic fatigue.

Social Support

CFS patients often encounter poor understanding and inadequate awareness of CFS by healthcare professionals and the public. This compounds the problems faced by CFS patients, including children. Moreover, others lose support from family and friends due to the popular misperception that CFS "isn't real."[21] Professional caregivers must then broaden their services to include briefing the people close to the patient about the need for understanding.

Studies have found that improvement in people with CFS was associated with social support.[22] They also found that during the year before the onset of CFS, people acknowledged less social support than healthy controls.[23] This is in line with the detrimental effects of social disengagement, but this time, the disconnection was on the part of people around the patient. Moreover, CFS is linked with an individual's overall happiness, including his relationships with loved ones and coworkers, as well as other social aspects outside the family.

People around the patient must fathom the CFS patient's circumstances when interacting with him. All of this is key to maintaining good collaborative relationships aimed at improving the patient's health.

HOW TO DEAL WITH CFS-RELATED STRESS

One common indicator of life-threatening stress is post-traumatic stress disorder (PTSD). Somatic complaints of CFS were thought to enhance the stress disorder. Experts have asserted that CFS might have been triggered by deployment-related stress. The study involves 15,000 former Gulf War soldiers and 15,000 other veterans who completed questionnaires evaluating their exposure to possible risks, potential variables, their functional impairments, and their medical past. The questionnaire included the somatic symptoms prevalent in previous patients.[24]

From the data collected, researchers found that the level of stress varies based on the deployment of the veterans. Those who aren't utilized in warfare have minimal stress; reservists deployed to a location away from the Persian Gulf possess moderate stress; and those deployed to the Gulf have the highest levels of stress. The demographics were analyzed, and the groups that had post-traumatic stress disorder or CFS-like illnesses were compared. The veterans demonstrating positivity in spite of post-traumatic stress are mainly older nonwhite females in the enlisted ranks in the Army and National Guard. Soldiers who are positive for CFS-like illness tend to be younger, single, and enlisted in the reserves. The prevalence of traumatic stress was found to range from 3.3 to 22.6 percent.[25]

The correlation between post-traumatic stress or CFS-like illness and the development of full-blown diagnosed CFS has been proven. Stressor intensity affects the rate of post-traumatic stress. From here, it's argued that post-traumatic stress leads to the stress-related behavioral problems in chronic fatigue syndrome. The rate is substantially higher in conflicts where stressor intensity is greater. When related to combat, the rate of CFS-like illness didn't change significantly for Gulf War veterans. Deployment stress relates to the onset of CFS in a veteran population. However, scientists can't be assured that other elements specific to serving in the Gulf might have contributed to the accelerated rates of CFS among Gulf War veterans. Aside from this, there are no other studies that relate the occurrence of CFS with stress, though the latter is an established indicator of the former. Stressor intensity is pertinent when studying the medical aftermath of stress, which plays a relatively minor role in CFS in the Gulf environment.[26]

In the workplace, employers need to make adjustments for workers with CFS; to do otherwise, they risk compromising work quality. The symptoms brought about by CFS may also affect employee evaluations. Employers and superiors must be patient with workers suffering with CFS. Moreover, society ought to be cognizant of such a syndrome in order to employ psychiatric maneuvers that can often impose on the physical well-being of the patient. Someone who cannot work because of a disorder is at risk for depression, which is needless when solutions for dealing with CFS are available. Lastly, solidarity and camaraderie among coworkers are needed to address the occupation-related effects of CFS.[27]

Positive Mood

As in the case of office culture, work efficiency and effectiveness is reliant upon how well people work with tiredness, and having a positive mood only makes things better. This is where drive and motivation comes in—drive and motivation should be as pervasive as the illness. When organs deteriorate, all that's left is the mind fervently believing that the body still can go on. It means striving for happiness through optimism—unless the person prefers rotting away with the illness. If a patient is already sick, expelling negative thoughts can only help.[28]

A low mood can result in further exhaustion. When a CFS patient feels downcast to the point of moroseness around others, mood regulation should be employed with care. Asking others to try to understand him might be a form of straightforward communication that assists everyone in adjusting to interactions with him.

ANALYSIS

Mental state has been found to predict health outcomes, and the mind and body form a fascinating and indeed powerful link. It's amazing how serenity or doom can spring from a material organ such as the brain.

13

COLLECTIVE EFFORTS

As this comprehensive discussion about chronic fatigue syndrome (CFS) nears its end, patients and caregivers should know that CFS has a huge impact on the community and society in general, since it largely affects the productivity and the ability of an individual to work and fully function, as well as to execute routines of daily life. The disorder also causes financial hardship to those afflicted, which is all related to the decreased productivity of the affected population.[1] In recent years, governments have played a substantial role in the advocacy and treatment of CFS.[2]

WHY THE GOVERNMENT NEEDS TO GET MORE INVOLVED

Millions of people are affected by CFS in the United States, and documents have stated that affected individuals endure long-term, chronic, debilitating, and incapacitating mental and physical pain, as well as aftereffects of fatigue that don't respond to rest. The fatigue is worsened by physical and mental stress or exertion, which diminishes the individual's capability to concentrate and causes impaired memory, tiredness and lethargy, and sleep disturbances. CFS patients must also deal with extensive diagnostic tests and clinical assessments that bear on their productivity at work and cause additional healthcare-related expenses. Again, all the above is why chronic fatigue syndrome can't be eradicated without a collective effort.[3]

Some patients with CFS might ask what their healthcare profession-al can do to help them. Even though the cause of chronic fatigue syn-drome hasn't been identified, healthcare professionals can offer pallia-tive treatment or treat the symptoms stemming from the disorder.[4] Informing the healthcare professional about the specific symptoms the patient experiences is an important step, since many of these symptoms can be treated. The healthcare professional can also recommend sup-port groups and other therapies tailored to the CFS sufferer that can help him cope with the condition.

Another question that frequently comes to mind is why the symp-toms of CFS seem to come and go. Although CFS can persist for years at a time, studies (some are funded by governments) indicate that chronic fatigue syndrome isn't classified as a progressive condition due to its cognitive symptoms.[5] The worst symptoms tend to occur during the first two years, after which the symptoms stabilize but persist chron-ically, wax and wane, or finally improve. Symptoms are unique to each patient involved, and the course of chronic fatigue syndrome can't be predicted. Yet another reason why government needs to get involved.[6]

Healthcare professionals diagnose CFS based on the client's symp-toms and medical history, as well as through diagnostic tests used to rule out other clinical anomalies. At present, there's no known cure for chronic fatigue syndrome and there is not a surefire treatment for the disorder itself; amelioration of the individual symptoms is the treat-ment. Most CFS patients fully recover from the disorder, and a few partially recover yet still experience symptoms, since clinical indicators may persist for years. Some CFS sufferers may experience periodic relapse, and since little is known regarding the actual cause of the disorder, the course of the disorder can't be determined in large-scale populations. Governments can assist in that regard.[7]

Chronic fatigue syndrome isn't contagious, and there's no known data indicating that it can be transferred from one individual to another. Barring viral implications, it can't be transmitted by contact, airborne droplet, blood transfusion, or other modes of diffusion, so there's no need to isolate patients diagnosed with chronic fatigue syndrome. Should governments get involved in the effort to find a cure, the need for emergency quarantine will not be of concern.

Chronic fatigue syndrome limits the individual's ability to work and stay productive in both home and the workplace, and it impairs the person's ability to participate fully in their daily activities. Hence, this condition tends to cause absenteeism from work, which may then lead to lost hours or even unemployment. Governments should take that into consideration. With fewer productive work periods, an individual's earnings would also decrease, resulting in less spending power or decreased earnings with which to support himself. This also causes a burden on the employers as well as family members due to unresolved conflicts that can arise because of the condition.[8]

CFS affects not only the diagnosed individuals and their families, but also their workplace, relationships, community, and society in general. Fewer productive employees means a decline in the labor force, which causes a decline in work that tends to have a negative impact on both employer and employee. A healthier population is more efficient, performing tasks on time, delivering positive work performance, generating more revenue for businesses and corporations, and ensuring the success of their companies. Ultimately, with the government receiving more taxpayer funds, improvements in the care of CFS would commence.[9]

HOW CORPORATIONS CAN HELP

Support Groups

The importance of support groups for chronic fatigue syndrome can't be overemphasized. No one is alone with the affliction, and recuperation is a collective effort: first, by ensuring the full cooperation of the individual and the desire to get well and to overcome the disorder, and second through the collective efforts of corporations, including nonprofits, and public awareness regarding the implications of CFS. Managing the symptoms of CFS is a struggle, but the cooperation and participation of companies helps significantly.

Agencies and Nonprofit Organizations Aimed at Eradicating CFS

Today, there's no known cure for CFS, although palliative options can help alleviate its symptoms. Treatments for CFS depend on the person's symptoms, as well as the prognosis and early detection of the disease. Research has been done in the United States and abroad to develop advanced treatments for chronic fatigue syndrome, as well as to document the neurological, immunological, cardiovascular, and respiratory effects on CFS patients. Such experiments have been funded by various nonprofit agencies such as those mentioned in the following paragraphs.

National Fibromyalgia Association (NFA)

Established in 1997, the NFA supports people diagnosed with fibromyalgia as well as other disorders related to pain symptoms, such as CFS. Its mission is to develop programs dedicated to improving the quality of life of the patients suffering from these diseases.[10]

National Fibromyalgia Research Association

National Fibromyalgia Research Association is an organization that funds research and continuing education for physicians and other healthcare workers. It organizes efforts in raising public awareness about the causes, early detection, prevention, and treatment of fibromyalgia. It has also produced a fibromyalgia exercise and fitness video, as well as fibromyalgia bracelets to raise awareness and garner support from the general public.[11]

International Association for CFS/ME

International Association for CFS/ME is a private organization that primarily aims to boost research and awareness for CFS. The group also advocates education regarding patient care, early discernment, and treatment. It conducts regular conferences with other groups to promote and evaluate research regarding the disorder and to strengthen efforts to decode it. This organization also runs seminars to educate doctors and other healthcare workers about treatment for patients.[12]

HHV-6 Foundation

HHV-6 Foundation is an entity that encourages research and the exchange of information among researchers and scientists in order to acquire grants to uphold research. One of its first advocacies was to determine the difference between an active and latent infection, as well as biological ciphers in the individuals diagnosed with CFS. The name HHV-6 stands for human herpesvirus 6, which many believe to be linked to chronic fatigue syndrome and pain-related symptoms.[13]

National Institute for Health and Care Excellence

National Institute for Health and Care Excellence is a British agency that advises individual treatment programs that prioritize maintaining optimum physical functions and abilities of the individual as well as strengthening emotional support, managing the symptoms of the condition, and raising public awareness of CFS.[14]

Organizations for CFS Education

PANDORA

PANDORA is an advocacy group that's one of the most active in fighting chronic fatigue syndrome through education and awareness regarding the prevention of CFS. This organization is located in Miami and was founded in 2007.[15]

Rocky Mountain CFIDS and FMS Association

Rocky Mountain CFIDS and FMS Association is an institute that maintains a website and online forums that provide education regarding CFS. They also offer practicums on its prevention and treatment.[16]

Wisconsin Chronic Fatigue Syndrome Association

Wisconsin Chronic Fatigue Syndrome Association is one of the first organizations supporting CFS education. They publish newsletters that offer information and updates about the disorder. They also host discussion forums as well as support services via phone, where people can talk to someone regarding their concerns about the syndrome.[17]

HOW CFS PATIENTS CAN HELP EACH OTHER

Since CFS itself is a formidable enemy, the CFS patient community should possess a strong community support network. Patient-to-patient groups provide information, research, encouragement, and support services to people suffering from the condition. They rally around relevant issues, such as the social and medical implications of labeling CFS as a medical and psychiatric form of disorder. They're the ones who push through studies in order to gain untarnished understanding of the medical condition. There are countless sites in the Internet promoting self-help and patient advocacy for this syndrome. After all, who can better help CFS patients than those who have suffered CFS themselves?[18]

Individuals diagnosed with chronic fatigue syndrome help each other by offering encouragement in promoting lifestyle changes.[19] Lifestyle changes are an most important aspect for a good prognosis since CFS hinders most patients in ways that cause both physical and emotional burdens. Through encouragement and patronage from fellow CFS patients, they can make their lives more enjoyable. Promoting rest as well as learning different stress-relieving techniques also helps the patient, because most suffer from extreme fatigue and nonrevitalizing sleep. Dietary modification—eating healthy foods in appropriate amounts—is also important, greatly improving the overall nutrition and well-being of the patient. Taking cooking classes or joining diet or weight-loss groups with other CFS sufferers is a good activity to support others and to promote companionship. People with CFS can also attend counseling sessions together, where healthcare professionals provide activities that help CFS patients to express their emotions and to share stories and experiences. Attending counseling sessions with other CFS patients allows one to explore sound coping strategies and also to learn how other people are surviving their disorder.[20]

Another way CFS patients can support each other is through use of an "energy diary" or journal. Logging activities as well as noting thoughts and feelings help identify the times of the day and activities that trigger stress or fatigue. This also helps to confirm the CFS patient's activities during the day and documents certain patterns of the disorder as well as the factors contributing to increased fatigue and other symptoms such as headaches and muscle weakness. Through the use of an energy diary, a CFS patient is also able to effectively schedule his activities—such as taking naps at predetermined times—and to identify stressors to eradicate from his daily routine. [21]

Individuals with CFS can also support each other by attending relaxation and meditation classes. Through relaxation and meditation, patients learn to scope out the situations that they find psychologically and physically stressful, as well as the activities that help them to handle these different stressors. A healthcare provider may create an exercise plan for the group. Most CFS patients experience fatigue easily, even as a result of moderate exercise, so the healthcare professional should start with light exercises and gradually increase the intensity according to each patient's ability. Group moderators can also provide patients evaluations at each week's end to identify areas of improvement. [22]

Support among patients with CFS, such as meetings and discussion groups, helps lessen the possibility of developing depression or other mental health–related disorders. Since CFS is a debilitating, long-term condition, CFS sufferers in some cases may develop depression due to decreased physical activity, inability to work, and lack of support from friends or family members. Although there are certain medications for treating depression, such as SSRIs, being able to express and communicate feelings and to articulate emotions and stressful experiences to someone else decreases the chances of developing depression, especially in patients with CFS. [23] Another way CFS sufferers can support each other is to encourage each other to follow the course of treatment advocated by their physician and other healthcare professionals. [24]

CFS Patients Helping Each Other to Deal with Stress

People have their own ways of shoring up against stress. Some studies show that stress can cause excessive eating or other unhealthy habits. Research demonstrates that a healthier way to deal with stress is through exercise, healthier eating habits, and more effective ways in dealing with stressful situations, coupled with support from family and friends. [25]

CFS patients can help each other identify potential stressors and consider ways to cope with the disorder effectively. Group exercises are a fun way of supporting each other. Not only does exercise burn calories, but it also produces biochemicals known to counter the negative effect of cortisol, a stress hormone mentioned in an earlier chapter of this book. Exercise also helps control the blood's insulin and glucose levels. A minimum of twenty to thirty minutes of exercise each day, two or three times a week is recommended. Collaborative exercise is indispensible, but it's important to be careful not to overexert, since this may lead to increased cortisol levels, which is harmful to one's health. [26]

Classes that CFS patients could attend together include relaxation exercises, such as meditation sessions or yoga, deep-breathing courses, or guided imagery classes, wherein the patient would learn about ways to relax body and mind—a healthy way to deal with all types of stress. Some of these classes, often moderated by a CFS patient, teach participants to possess a sea of calmness wherein the body and mind are free from external stressors. This helps the patient develop his own relaxation and meditation techniques. [27]

Baking and cooking sessions are also activities in which CFS patients can enroll together, since from-scratch, homemade foods are healthier than processed foods, which are known to contain harmful chemicals that aren't the best for the patient's health. CFS patients could also collectively help each other by encouraging each other in breaking bad habits, such as smoking and alcohol consumption, which are known to increase cortisol levels and subsequently increase feelings of stress, lethargy, tiredness, and muscle weakness. [28]

ANALYSIS

Much like other chronic disorders and debilitating conditions, CFS accounts for a large portion of personal, medical, as well as healthcare-related economic costs. That's partially why the dilemma of CFS should be addressed collectively. As is the case with other conditions such as cardiovascular diseases, diabetes mellitus, and cancer, government agencies have spearheaded funding and organized advocacy groups to raise public awareness and support.

14

CONCLUSION

Time and again, humanity is pushed to the brink of its limits. Here comes another complex disorder with devastating ramifications, the origins of which remain shadowy. Despite the efforts of healthcare professionals, definitive treatment of chronic fatigue syndrome (CFS) remains elusive.[1] By now, the reader should understand that what makes CFS even more difficult is the diagnosis—it's almost impossible to self-diagnose, and help from experts is uncertain, as its symptoms are rampant in many other medical disorders. Studies revealed that in the United States, less than 20 percent of the estimated four million people with CFS have been diagnosed.[2]

HOPE DESPITE THE DAMAGING NATURE OF CFS

So, what more is there to do? Will it be to despair over one's current helplessness or to continue working harder? There's nothing wrong in hoping for better. Hope is what keeps individuals moving forward. Continuing studies and clinical surveys will provide the most accurate test for the diagnosis of CFS, as well as the most effective treatment. As experts note, there has been progress in understanding the nature and management of CFS over the years as more countries, researchers, and clinicians have become involved. Therefore, there's much reason for hope, which is perhaps the most beautiful thing in this world. Indeed, recovery starts with hope.[3]

It All Starts Here

Nowadays, many advancements have been made. In fact, progress is a never-ending process. Humans have an insatiable hunger for unraveling mysteries and making discoveries. They seek infinite answers from their inestimable questions. However, there are still many things beyond clear understanding, just like CFS. Looking back, where does anything really start? Long before Neil Armstrong landed on the moon, he may have struggled first learning to balance on his bike.

Surely, this is similar to understanding CFS. The disorder began hobbling people without their least knowledge of it. It's no wonder it was years before this condition was identified. Nonetheless, because of its continual recurrence, it was finally given a clear-cut definition by the Centers for Disease Control in 1994 as an unexplained, persistent, or relapsing fatigue of six months duration that can't be explained by other medical conditions.[4]

This was a major breakthrough, and since then, research followed suit. Currently, it can be said that scientists are attempting to fully decipher the nature of CFS and provide the definitive medication for it. That's why there's no place for anxiety. Everything will fall into position as long as hope and courage are in the driver's seat.[5]

Mystery of the Day: What's Really There to Hope For?

Chronic fatigue syndrome poses four major challenges. First, it's a major disorder. Second, it's not well known or understood by the general public. Although unfamiliar, it's not uncommon.[6] Third, its cause is still unknown, so prevention isn't foolproof. Fourth, there's still no official therapy, medicines, or treatment used today by healthcare professionals. Perhaps the greatest challenge posed by CFS is that it's very difficult to diagnose in a person without professional assistance.

The good news is that it's not as bad as it sounds. There's no standard treatment, but the medical community has developed several strategies based on the severity of a patient's CFS. Addressing the challenge in diagnosis, numerous different studies are simultaneously working on providing better case definitions and encouraging professional caregivers from around the world to take up the challenge that CFS brings to the table. Raising awareness may be challenging at this point, but as long as there are different organizations and companies that continue to nurture concern, worldwide awareness of CFS may be achieved.[7]

The cause of CFS is still undetermined but several theories are already in line. Persistence and patience link the doctors specializing in CFS, and it's almost certain that the exact cause will be discovered eventually. Also, cures are elusive for many disorders, although their causes may have long been identified. The point being that pinpointing the source of CFS won't automatically eradicate it. Right now, the process of interpreting the mystery of CFS is already underway.

It's All There

When does consistent and sincere hard work really end? Today, it's apparent that there's still a lot of light to be shed on the gloom of CFS but all that's to be done is to keep moving forward. CFS is a disorder about to be cracked wide open.

IMPORTANCE OF SEEKING PROFESSIONAL HELP

Every patient needs the courage to stand up and take on the challenges of his disorder. However, he also needs the help of a healthcare professional to diagnose and prescribe a course of treatment. Self-examination is one of the best things a patient can do for himself, but self-examination is only the start. It's usually ineffective to examine oneself without consulting a doctor, leaving the management of the disorder to hearsay.[8]

It's like playing darts with a blindfold; the target is there, but it can't be seen. Nothing beats proper diagnosis from professionals. Medical-based approaches offer more accurate diagnoses and treatments. From there, the patient is poised to get healthier.[9]

Better to Be Safe than Sorry

With one's health at stake, CFS patients should never take symptoms for granted. A mild fever could be the result of malaria, while a simple string of infections can indicate bone cancer. Alternative and substandard medication can lessen or perhaps resolve an ailment but not in the long run. What's even worse: as people keep relying on these short-term remedies, eventually they lose effectiveness. It's therefore highly recommended that prescribers oversee treatments for patients with CFS. Investment in health is the best wager of all.[10]

When Darkness Gets Darker

Many questions still surround chronic fatigue syndrome in the medical world. As stated by experts, CFS patients have great variability in their reactions to treatments.[11] Finding treatments and dosages that help is by trial and error. Since even experts have yet to arrive at a definitive treatment, CFS patients must rely on their expertise all the more. The concept is simple: don't swing a hammer at a rock that even a backhoe can't break. Taking matters into one's own hands comes into play after getting guidelines from the doctor. Treatment doesn't end inside the hospital or clinic; it continues into the patient's day-to-day life.

THE IMPORTANCE OF PATIENCE AND CONFIDENCE

Optimism and consistency are important for patients with any type of disability. Before one can do something, he first has to *believe* that he can do it. Moreover, he has to maintain his belief that he can do it. These characteristics, together with the wonders of science, ensure a bright outlook for patients. But without a clear understanding of the disorder, patients diagnosed with CFS should seek appropriate profes-sional medical help. The bigger the impediment, the more help and belief one must possess in order to overcome it.[12]

Getting Better through Patience

In a strange way, simply knowing that one has CFS is something for which to be thankful. A patient diagnosed with CFS has already over-come one hurdle: the diagnosis of the disorder remains difficult even among professionals. With a firm diagnosis, the CFS patient can obtain appropriate therapy and medication. However, how long recovery takes remains uncertain. CFS symptoms vary in degree, and although there are many cases in which improvement was reported, no single definitive therapy or treatment has been uncovered by medical experts. One can only bear with it and trust that the condition will be subdued sooner or later. [13]

Having the Confidence to Cope

It's not impossible for people with CFS to improve their health and quality of life. Several self-care strategies have been laid out for them. Physically, one must live a healthy lifestyle that includes exercise, a balanced diet, and restful sleep. He must pay attention to and take action for his health. The paradox is that strenuous exercise often makes CFS symptoms worse, but people with the syndrome must exercise in order to feel more energetic. So what should be done? Several studies proved that activities such as aerobic exercise and other low-impact activities can improve the nervous system function of people with CFS. [14]

Generally, the key is to balance and pace the workouts: they should never be beyond one's capacity but beneficial enough to improve one's physical condition. Healthcare professionals can suggest specific therapies based on the degree of the patient's CFS, which should give the patient confidence in coping with CFS. [15]

ANALYSIS

In the final analysis, denying CFS of its wrathful onslaughts truly depends on the willpower of the sufferer. Patience and confidence are important characteristics, but the reader should also remember that it's not impossible for people with CFS to improve the health and quality of their lives. After all, only amid darkness is the brightest lamp sought.

GLOSSARY

acetylcholinesterase: An enzyme that carries out the process of breakdown of acetylcholine (a neurotransmitter) in the region between two nerve cells (the synaptic cleft) in order to transmit impulses from one neuron to another.

achalasiacardia: Also called cardiospasm. In this case, it's the neuro-muscular failure of esophagus relaxation, especially at its lower end.

actin-myosin cross bridging: Responsible for the force generation and contraction of skeletal muscle. Certain myosin-binding sites present on actin that bond with myosin, forming cross bridges, which is an important step in skeletal muscle contraction.

adenine: One of the four nucleic acid bases derived from purine. It combines with thymine to form the double-stranded DNA.

adenosinediphosphate (ADP): An organic compound that is essential for the process of metabolism. One molecule of ADP is composed of one molecule of adenine combined with two molecules of phosphate on a sugar base.

adenosine triphosphate: A nucleotide with three phosphate groups that is regarded as the currency unit of energy in a cell.

adrenal androgens dehydroepiandrosterone (DHEA): A steroid hormone produced by the adrenal cortex that in females is responsible for control of processes like growth of pubic or axillary hair and maintenance of female sex drive.

agranulocytosis: A condition in which granulocyte counts decrease. The granulocytes are neutrophils, basophils, and eosinophils.

alpha-intrusion: Alpha waves are a kind of brain wave that originate from the occipital lobe primarily when a person is awake and relaxing but has closed his eyes. Alpha-intrusion occurs when a person generates alpha waves during non-REM sleep.

anemia: A condition in which the number of the red blood cells or the amount of hemoglobin decreases. It can also be explained as the reduced capacity of oxygen transport.

arrhythmia: Irregular heartbeat.

arthralgias: Joint pain.

autoantibodies: Antibodies produced by one's body as an immune response to destroy one's own specific proteins.

autonomic nervous system: A part of the peripheral nervous system that is responsible for involuntary responses like digestion, salivation, heart rate, and breathing.

axis 1 disorders: These disorders fall under the category of psychiatric disorders and include anxiety disorders, mood disorders, eating and psychotic disorders, as well as dissociative and substance use disorders.

biomarker: A biological indicator—a molecule, gene, or simply a characteristic trait—that primarily is used to study various aspects of a disease or a biological condition like the onset of disease and its progress, how well it is responding to treatment measures, and so on.

bursae: A closed, fluid-filled sac lined with a synovial membrane that is usually found in regions of friction, such as in an area where the tendon rubs against the bone.

cancer cachexia: A multifactorial syndrome that has characteristic features like anorexia and loss of appetite resulting in wasting of body tissues, atrophy of skeletal muscles, and immunity-related problems.

catalysis: The process altering (increasing or decreasing) the velocity of a chemical reaction in the presence of a compound (catalyst) that doesn't get used up during the process.

cavernosal arteries: These are deep blood vessels in the penis that supply blood to the corpora cavernosa and aid in erection.

chromosomes: Chromosomes are present within the nucleus of a cell and carry the genetic information that is passed on from parents to their children.

ciliary beating: Cilia are thin extensions that line various body parts like the trachea and fallopian tubes. They move in a beating manner to thrust out dirt and dust (as in the case of the trachea) and transport ovum to ovary (in the case of Fallopian tubes).

creatinine: A chemical waste product of muscles that's used for measuring kidney health.

cushingoid: Describes the features of a Cushing's syndrome or Cushing's disease, such as excessive facial hair, striations on the trunk, and pads of fat on face and upper part of back.

cytomegalovirus: A group of herpesviruses that have mild or no significant effects on a normal healthy person but that can create serious complications in fetuses, patients who have undergone organ transplantation, and those with HIV.

dysautonomia: When the autonomic nervous system isn't functioning properly.

dysmenorrhea: Painful menstruation.

dysphoria: Diffuse uneasiness with life.

dyspnea: Shortness of breath or difficulty breathing due to lung or heart problems.

endergonic: Any reaction that requires external energy to progress.

endocrine system: The system of glands that are responsible for controlling metabolism and other physiological processes through the secretion of hormones into blood circulation.

enterocolitis: Inflammation of the colon and small intestine.

epidemiology: The science in which various aspects of a disease process like the incidence and pattern of distribution is dealt with.

ergosterol: A sterol produced by yeasts that undergoes conversion to form vitamin D12 under ultraviolet rays.

exergonic: Any reaction that causes the release of energy into the external environment.

ex-vivo: That which happens outside the organism's body.

gastroesophageal junction: Also known as cardia, this is the junction between the distal part of the esophagus and the proximal part of the stomach.

gastrointestinal mucosa: The innermost layer of the gastrointestinal tract, which that has three layers: epithelium, lamina propria, and muscularis mucosa.

glial cell: A cell that forms the neuroglia like astrocutes and microglia.

granulomatous disease: Any disease in which the growth of minute blood vessels and connective tissue can be observed.

hematopoiesis: The creation and development of blood cells inside the body.

homeoregulatory: Involving the regulation of body temperature.

homeostasis: The tendency of the body to maintain a state of equilibrium by regulating various physiological processes within the body.

hospitalists: Medical professionals or physicians who take care of the medical needs of hospitalized patients.

hypochondriacal: Related to hypochondria, or phobia or anxiety regarding one's health in which an individual suspects or fears that he is suffering from a grave illness.

hypocortisolism: Also known as adrenal insufficiency, a condition in which the adrenal glands fail to produce enough steroid hormones.

hypoperfusion: The reduced flow of blood through any organ.

hypotension: Blood pressure lower than the normal range.

interferons: Glycoproteins that are released from animal cells as an immune response and can inhibit the replication process in viruses.

interleukins: Cytokines produced by leukocytes for immune response regulation.

intracellular: That which occurs within a cell.

mitochondria: Cytoplasmic organelles that are spherical or rod shaped and are referred to as the powerhouses of a cell, as they are concerned with ATP synthesis.

mycoplasmapneumonia: An infectious disease that occurs in children and adults and is caused by mycoplasma pneumonia. Since the disease affects the lungs, the symptoms generally include fever, cough, and upper respiratory infection.

nondiscocytes: Abnormal and less flexible red blood cells that lack the typical disc shape of a red blood cell and that occur due to magnesium deficiency.

non-REM sleep: Of the five stages of sleep, non-REM sleep comprises stages one through four and is characterized by reduced heart and breathing rates, decreased metabolic activity, and an absence of dreaming.

osteoporosis: A disease that causes the formation of porous bones due to excessive loss of proteins as well as minerals like calcium.

pathophysiology: The study of the ways that the normal functions of the body get disrupted due to disease process.

perfusion: The process of fluid passage through any organ, such as the heart.

peripheral nervous system: One of the two major nervous systems of the body that forms a link between the central nervous system and the sensory organs.

pharyngitis: Inflammation of the pharynx characterized by symptoms like sore throat.

phonasthenia: Difficulty experienced during voice production due to factors like fatigue.

photosynthesis: A chemical process occurring in green plants in which carbon dioxide and water in the presence of sunlight are converted into carbohydrates.

physiological: Related to the physiology or the normal functioning of any living organism.

phytochemicals: A class of chemicals naturally found in plants.

postural orthostatic tachycardia syndrome (POTS): The condition in which the heart rate shoots up abnormally when a person stands in an upright position.

psychosocial: Psychological and social.

psychosomatic: Anything pertaining to the interaction of the body and mind.

school avoidance behavior: A type of anxiety diorder seen in children when they refuse to go to school due to various reasons like separation anxiety or depression.

somatic nervous system: A division of the peripheral nervous system responsible for all the body's voluntary movements by conveying impulses from central nervous system to skeletal muscles and vice versa.

Stevens-Johnson syndrome: A form of erythema multiforme that occurs as an allergic reaction to certain drugs. It is a fatal condition in which the person has symptoms like flu and red rash all over the body that become painful blisters.

temporomandibular joint (TMJ) disorder: A disorder affecting the temporomandibular joint, which is located between the mandible and the skull, with symptoms that include jaw pain and pain in the adjoining muscles.

tonsiliar: Related to tonsils, a collection of lymphatic tissues present at various sites of the body and named accordingly. For instance, palatine tonsils are at the back of the mouth.

urticaria: An allergic response of the body to some food or medicines that is represented by the presence of itchy skin at various places on the body.

ventilatory failure: Type II respiratory failure in which the ventilator process is hampered and the carbon dioxide produced by the body isn't excreted adequately.

APPENDIX A

Chronic Fatigue Syndrome–Related Links

- www.betterhealth.vic.gov.au/bhcv2/bhcarticles.nsf/pages/Chronic_fatigue_syndrome
- www.bupa.co.uk/individuals/health-information/directory/c/hi-chronic-fatigue-syndrome
- www.cdc.gov/cfs/
- www.cfids-cab.org/MESA/ccpccd.pdf
- http://chealth.canoe.ca/condition_info_details.asp?disease_id=32
- www.co-cure.org/MEICC.pdf
- www.dailymail.co.uk/health/article-2006038/Myalgic-encephalomyelitis-caused-virus.html
- www.fm-cfs.ca/
- http://guidance.nice.org.uk/CG53
- www.hfme.org/whatisme.htm
- www.hhs.gov/advcomcfs/
- http://jnm.snmjournals.org/content/early/2014/03/21/jnumed.113.131045.abstract
- http://kidshealth.org/parent/system/ill/cfs.html
- www.mayoclinic.org/diseases-conditions/chronic-fatigue-syndrome/
- www.meassociation.org.uk
- www.mecfs.org.au/what-is-meorcfs
- http://medical-dictionary.thefreedictionary.com/Myalgic+encephalitis

- www.medscape.com/viewarticle/773334
- www.name-us.org/
- www.ncbi.nlm.nih.gov/books/NBK53577/
- www.netdoctor.co.uk/diseases/facts/cfs_managing_003805.htm
- www.nhs.uk/conditions/Chronic-fatigue-syndrome
- www.nlm.nih.gov/medlineplus/chronicfatiguesyndrome.html
- http://onlinelibrary.wiley.com/doi/10.1111/j.1365-2796.2011.02428.x/full
- www.patient.co.uk/doctor/chronic-fatigue-syndrome
- www.sciencedaily.com/news/health_medicine/chronic_fatigue_syndrome/
- www.thegracecharityforme.org/what.asp

APPENDIX B

Chronic Fatigue Syndrome Research and Training

Alison Hunter Memorial
Foundation
PO Box 6132
North Sydney NSW 2059
Australia
+61 2 9958 6285
www.ahmf.org

Associated New Zealand ME
Society
PO Box 36-307, Northcote
Auckland, New Zealand
+64 (09) 269 6374
www.anzmes.org.nz

Autoimmunity Research
Foundation
3423 Hill Canyon Ave.
Thousand Oaks, CA 91360
(818) 584-1201
foundation@
autoimmunityresearch.org

www.autoimmunityresearch.org

California Capital CFIDS
Association
PO Box 660362
Sacramento, CA 95866
(916) 484-3788
CalcapitalCFIDS@bigfoot.com
http://ottem.org/ccca

CFIDS Association of America
6827 Colony on Fairview Dr.
Charlotte, NC 28210
(704) 364-0016
http://solvecfs.org

CFS Research Foundation
2 The Briars
Sarratt, Rickmansworth
Hertfordshire WD3 6AU, United
Kingdom
+44 (0)192 326 8641

http://cfsrf.org.uk/

Chronic Fatigue Research and
Treatment Unit at King's College
London
Mapother House, 1st Floor
De Crespigny Park
Denmark Hill
London, United Kingdom SE5
8AZ
+44 (0)203 228 5075
Fax: +44 (0)203 228 5074
www.kcl.ac.uk/innovation/groups/
projects/cfs/index.aspx

Chronic Fatigue Syndrome,
Fibromyalgia & Chemical
Sensitivity Coalition of Chicago
PO Box 277
Wilmette, IL 60091
(773) 650-1332
www.cfccc.net

Chronic Pain and Fatigue
Research Center at University of
Michigan Health System
24 Frank Lloyd Wright Dr.
Ann Arbor, MI 48106
(734) 998-6939
Fax: (734) 998-6900
www.med.umich.edu/painre-
search

The Connecticut CFIDS & FM
Association, Inc.
PO Box 3010
Milford, CT 06460
(800) 952-2037

www.ct-cfids-fm.org

FM-CFS Canada
310-1500 Bank Street
Ottawa, Ontario K1H 1B8
(877) 437-4673
office@fm-cfs.ca
http://fm-cfs.ca

International Association for
Chronic Fatigue Syndrome/ Myalgic Encephalomyelitis
27 N. Wacker Dr., Suite 416
Chicago, IL 60606
(847) 258-7248
Fax: (847) 579-0975
admin@iacfsme.org
www.iacfsme.org

Invest in ME
PO Box 561
Eastleigh SO50 0GQ
Hampshire
United Kingdom
+44 (0) 238 025 1719
Fax: +44 (0) 238 000 0040
www.investinme.org

Irish ME Trust
Carmichael House
North Brunswick Street
Dublin 7
00 353 1 401 3629
Fax: 00 353 1 401 3736
info@imet.ie
www.imet.ie

Massachusetts CFIDS/ME & FM
Association
PO Box 690305
Quincy, MA 02269
(617) 471-5559
www.masscfids.org

ME Association
7 Apollo Office Court
Radclive Road
Gawcott, Bucks MK18 4DF
United Kingdom
+44 (0)128 081 8964
admin@meassociation.org.uk
www.meassociation.org.uk

ME Research UK
The Gateway, North Methven St.
Perth PH1 5PP, United Kingdom
+44 (0)173 845 1234
editor@meresearch.org.uk

ME/CFS Australia Ltd.
2/240 Chapel Street
PRAHAN VIC 3181
+61 (03) 9529 1344
www.mecfs.org.au

ME/CFS Foreningen
Radhustorvet 1, 1
Sal 3520 Farum
44 95 97 00
mail@me-cfs.dk
www.me-cfs.dk

ME/CFS Society WA
The Centre for Neurological
Support

The Niche, 11 Aberdare Road
Nedlands, Perth
Western Australia 6009
+61 (08) 9346 7477
Fax: +61 (08) 9346 7534
www.mecfswa.org.au

ME/CFS/FM Support Association
Qld Inc.
St. Vincents Hospital
Scott Street, Toowoomba
Queensland 4350, Australia
+61 (07) 4632 8173
Fax: +61 (07) 4632 8173
www.mecfsfmq.org.au/

The National CFIDS Foundation
103 Aletha Rd.
Needham, MA 02492
(781) 449-3535
Fax: (781) 449-8606
info@ncf-net.org
www.ncf-net.org

New Jersey Chronic Fatigue
Syndrome Association, Inc.
PO Box 477
Florham Park, NJ 07932
(888) 835-3677
www.njcfsa.org

Nightingale Research Foundation
121 Iona St.
Ottawa Ontario K1Y 3M1
Canada
www.nigthingale.ca

Partnership for Research in CFS and ME (PRIME)
Minervation Ltd.
Salter's Boat Yard
Folly Bridge
Oxford OX1 4LB
www.prime-cfs.org

Simmaron Research Foundation
948 Incline Way
Incline Village, NV 89451
(775) 298-0030
Fax: (775) 298-0031
redefiningmecfs@gmail.com
http://simmaronresearch.org

Stanford Myalgic Encephalomye-
litis/Chronic Fatigue Syndrome
(ME/CFS) Initiative at Stanford
University of Medicine
291 Campus Drive Rm LK3C02

Li Ka Shing Building, 3rd floor
Stanford, CA 94305
(650) 725-3900
http://chronicfatigue.stanford.edu/

Whitmore Peterson Institute for
Neuro-Immune Disease at
University of Nevada
1664 N. Virginia St.
Reno, NV 89557
(775) 682-8250
Fax: +1 (775) 682-8258
info@wpinstitute.org
www.wpinstitute.org

Wisconsin ME/CFS Association,
Inc.
733 Lois Dr.
Sun Prairie, WI 53590
(608) 834-1001
www.wicfs-me.org

APPENDIX C

Chronic Fatigue Syndrome–Related Organizations

California Capital CFIDS
Association (CCCA)
PO Box 660362
Sacramento, CA 95866
(916) 484-3788
CalCapitalCFIDS@bigfoot.com
www.ottem.org

Central Virginia Chronic Fatigue
Syndrome and Fibromyalgia
Association
PO Box 5733
Charlottesville, VA 22905
(434) 984-3419
cfsfma@avenue.org
www.cfsfma.avenue.org

CFIDS Association of America
6827 Colony Fairview Dr.
Charlotte, NC 28210
(704) 364-0016
CFIDS@CFIDS.ORG

www.cfids.org

Chronic Fatigue Syndrome/
Fibromyalgia Organization
of Georgia, Inc.
1210 Wooten Lake Rd. NW
Kennesaw, GA 30144
(770) 974-0157
www.cfog.us

Chronic Syndrome Support
Association, Inc.
801 Riverside Drive
Lumberton, NC 28358
www.cssa-inc.org

Connecticut CFIDS & FM
Association, Inc.
PO Box 3010
Milford, CT 06460
(800) 952-2037
www.ct-cfids-fm.org

Fibromyalgia Network
PO Box 31750
Tucson, AZ 85751
(520) 290-5508
www.fmnetnews.com

International Association for CFS/
ME
27 N. Wacker Dr., Suite 416
Chicago, IL 60606
(847) 258-7248
Fax: (847) 579-0975
admin@iacfsme.org
www.iacfsme.org

Las Vegas Fibromyalgia/Chronic
Fatigue Syndrome Support Group
4308 Rosebank Circle
Las Vegas, NV 89108
(702) 647-4791
shebrews@yahoo.com

Massachusetts CFIDS/ME & FM
Association
PO Box 690305
Quincy, MA 02269
(617) 471-5559
www.masscfids.org

National CFIDS Foundation, Inc.
103 Aletha Rd.
Needham, MA 02492
(781) 449-3535
Fax: (781) 449-8606
info@ncf-net.org
www.ncf-net.org

National Fibromyalgia
Partnership, Inc.
140 Zinn Way
Linden, VA 22642
www.fmpartnership.org

New Jersey Chronic Fatigue
Syndrome Association, Inc.
PO Box 477
Florham Park, NJ 07932
(888) 835-3677
pegwalk@aol.com
www.njcfsa.org

Open Medicine Institute
2500 Hospital Dr., Bldg. 2
Mountain View, CA 94040
(650) 691-8633
Fax: (650) 644-3223
info@openmedicineinstitute.org
www.openmedicineinstitute.org

Organization for Fatigue &
Fibromyalgia Education & Research
1002 E. South Temple, Suite 408
Salt Lake City, UT 84102
support@OfferUtah.org
www.offerutah.org

Rocky Mountain CFS/ME & FM
Association
7020 E Girard Ave., Suite 207
Denver, CO 80224
(303) 423-7367
link@rmcfa.org
www.rmcfa.org

Wisconsin Myalgic Encephalom-
yelitis/Chronic Fatigue Syndrome
Association, Inc.
733 Lois Dr.

Sun Prairie, WI 53590
(608) 834-1001
www.wicfs-me.org

APPENDIX D

Nationally Recognized Chronic Fatigue Syndrome Clinics

Alternatives: A Center for
Conscious Health
11036 Oak St.
Rockbrook Village
Omaha, NE 68144
(402) 827-9450
Fax: (402) 827-9471
info@alternativesomaha.com
www.centerforconscioushealth
.com

Amen Clinic
1000 Marina Blvd.
Brisbane, CA, 94005
(650) 416-7830
Fax: (650) 871-8874
www.amenclinics.com

Annapolis Integrative Medicine
1819 Bay Ridge Ave., Suite 200
Annapolis, MD 21403

(410) 266-3613
Fax: (410) 266-6104
www.annapolisintegrative
medicine.com

Austin Family Practice
11410 Jolleyville Rd.
Austin, TX 78759
(512) 346-3637
www.robertthoresondo.com

Barrow Neurological Institute
350 West Thomas Rd.
Phoenix, AZ 85013
(602) 406-6281
www.thebarrow.org

Black Bear Naturopathic Clinic
2831 Fort Missoula Rd, Suite 105
Missoula, MT 59804
(406) 542-2147

Fax: (406) 728-0978
www.blackbearnaturopaths.com

Boston Medical Center
840 Harrison Ave.
Boston, MA 02118
(617) 638-8000
www.bmc.org

Caring Counselor
Boulder, CO 80304
(303) 413-8091
pat@caringcounselor.com
www.caringcounselor.com

Celebration of Health Association
122 Thurman St.
Bluffton, OH 45817
(800) 788-4627
Fax: (419) 358-1855
mail@healthcelebration.com
www.healthcelebration.com

Center for Integrative Medicine
81 Hall St., Suite 1
Concord, NH 03301
(603) 228-7600
www.cfim.org

Charles R. Meyers, LAC
Acupuncture and Traditional
Chinese Medicine
2 West Park St.
Lebanon, NH 03766
(603) 442-9535
chas@charlesmeyerstcm.com
www.charlesmeyerstcm.com

Cheney Clinic
80 Peachtree Rd., Suite 208
Asheville, NC 28803
(828) 274-6665
Fax: (828) 274-6917
ddamron@cheneyclinic.com
www.cheneyclinic.com

Choices Integrative Healthcare
95 Soldiers Pass Rd., Suite B
Sedona, AZ 86336
(928) 203-4844
www.choiceshealthcare.com

Chronic Fatigue Clinic
Stanford School of Medicine
300 Pasteur Dr.
Stanford, CA 94305
(650) 723-6961
Fax: (650) 725-8418
www.chronicfatigue.stanford.edu

Chronic Fatigue Clinic at
Harborview
Harborview Medical Center
325 Ninth Ave., 7th Floor, Maleng
Building
Seattle, WA 98104
(206) 520-5000
www.uwmedicine.org

Cleveland Clinic
9500 Euclid Ave.
Cleveland, OH 44195
(216) 444–2200
www.clevelandclinic.org

Combined Health Care

Professionals
5140 NE Antioch Rd.
Kansas City, MO 64119
(816) 453-5545
www.drnancy.com

Connecticut Center for Health
87 Bernie O'Rourke Dr.
Middletown, CT 06457
(860) 347-8600
Fax: (860) 347-8434
www.connecticutcenterforhealth.
com

Dakota Medical Clinic
3408 Dakota Ave. South
St. Louis Park, MN 55416
(952) 924-1053
Fax: (952) 924-0254
www.dakotamc.com

Dallas Neurological Associates
403 West Campbell Rd., Suite 400
Richardson, TX 75080
(972) 783-8900
Fax: (972) 644-7926
www.dallasneurological.com

Dr. George J. Juetersonke
LifePulse Practice
3525 American Dr.
Colorado Springs, CO 80917
(719) 597-6075
Fax: (719) 573-6529
www.juetersonke.com

Dr. Teitelbaum's Clinic

Benmere Rd.
Glen Burnie, MD 21060
(410) 573-5389
Fax: 410-590-3047
office@endfatigue.com
www.endfatigue.com

Environmental Health and
Allergy Center
11585 W Florissant Ave.
Florissant, MO 63033
(314) 921-5600
Fax: (314) 921-8273
ehacstl@ehacstl.com
www.ehacstl.com

Fatigue Clinic of Michigan
G3494 Beecher Rd.
Flint, MI 48522
(810) 230-8677
www.cfids.com

Fatigue Consultation Clinic
1002 E South Temple St., Suite
408
Salt Lake City, UT 84102
(801) 359-7400
Fax: (801) 359-7404
FatigueConsultationClin-
ic@gmail.com
www.fcclinic.com

Fibromyalgia and Chronic
Fatigue Syndrome: Life Balance
PO Box 583
Stony Brook, NY 11790
(516) 702-4213
info@lifebalance7.com

www.lifebalance7.com

Fibromyalgia Treatment &
Learning Center
650 University Ave., Suite 200
Sacramento, CA 95825
(916) 922-8400
www.fmtlc.com

Four Rivers Naturopathic Clinic,
PC
1449 Lincoln Way
Auburn, CA 95603
(530) 823-1335
www.fourriversclinic.com

Gordon Medical Associates
3471 Regional Parkway
Santa Rosa, CA 95403
(707) 575- 5180
Fax: (707) 575- 5509
info@gordonmedical.com
www.gordonmedical.com

Greenhouse Naturopathic
Medicine
Spruce Park Professional Center
109 Ponemah Road, Suite 9
Amherst, NH 03031
(603) 249-5771
Fax: (603) 249-5924
www.greenhousemedicine.com

GW Medical Faculty Associates
2150 Pennsylvania Ave., NW
Washington, DC 20037
(202) 741-3000
www.gwdocs.com

Healing Arts Medical Center
Heights Medical Tower
427 W 20th St., Suite 602
Houston, TX 77008
(713) 802-1177
Fax: (713) 802-1277
info@awakenhealth.com
www.awakenhealth.com

Health Equations
PO Box 323
Newfane, VT 05345
(802) 365-9213
Fax: (802) 365-9218
service@healthequations.com
www.healthequations.com

Health for Life
2302 Amstel Lane
Vista, CA 92084
(760) 586-2627
info@alternativehealthandhealing.
com
www.alternativehealthandhealing.
com

Hillside Center for Behavioral
Services
8435 Holly Rd.
Grand Blanc, MI 48439
(810) 424-2400
www.genesys.org

Huber Natural Health, LLC
289 Main St.
Salem, NH 03079
(603) 890-9900

info@hubernaturalhealth.com
www.hubernaturalhealth.com

Hunter-Hopkins Center
7421 Carmel Executive Park Dr.
Charlotte, NC 28226
(704) 543-9692
drlapp@drlapp.net
www.drlapp.com

Infinity Wellness Center
205 Wild Basin Road S, Suite 2B
Austin, TX 78746
(512) 328-0505
info@austinholisticdr.com
www.austinholisticdr.com

Integrative Chiropractor Beverly
Hills
60 S Beverly Dr.
Beverly Hills, CA 90212
(310) 282-8882
www.wholebodycures.com

Integrative Healing Center
403 Main St., Suite 1
Port Washington, NY 11050
(516) 676-0200
Fax: (516) 676-2809
www.getintegrativehealth.com

Integrative Health Care of
Winona
356 E Sarnia St.
Winona, MN 55987
(507) 457-9000
Fax: (507) 457-9001
frontdesk@karenvrchota.com

www.karenvrchota.com

Jace Wellness Center
10843 Magnolia Blvd., Suite 1
North Hollywood, CA 91601
(818) 505-8610
www.jacemedical.com

Jeanne Hubbuch Family Practice
124 Watertown St., #2F
Watertown, MA 02472
(617) 744-0401
Fax: (617) 744-5346
drhubbuch@aol.com
www.drhubbuch.com

Johns Hopkins Medicine
1800 Orleans St.
Baltimore, MD 21287
(410) 955-5000
www.hopkinsmedicine.org

Lester Clinic
3700 Thomas Rd., #207
Santa Clara, CA 95054
(408) 844-0010
lesterclinic@gmail.com
www.lesterclinic.com

Manhattan Integrative Medicine
841 Broadway, 60th St., Suite
1012
New York, NY 10023
(917) 261-3771
Fax: (212) 262-2416
www.davidborensteinmd.com

Mary Claire Wise, MD

Holistic Medicine
4138 W Henrietta Rd.
Rochester, NY 14623
(585) 334-8020
marywisemd@yahoo.com
www.drmarywise.com

Mayo Clinic
13400 E Shea Blvd.
Scottsdale, AZ 85259
(480) 301-8000
Fax: (480) 301-9310
www.mayoclinic.org

Minneapolis Clinic of Neurology
4225 Golden Valley Rd.
Golden Valley, MN 55422
(763) 588-0661
www.minneapolisclinic.com

Nathanael Medical Center
1435 W Main St.
Dothan, AL 36301
(334) 702-8872
www.nathanaelmedicalcenter.com

Natural Health Medical Center,
Inc.
4469 Redondo Beach Blvd.
Lawndale, CA 90260
(310) 479-2266
Fax: (310) 479-2044
drhoang@naturalhealthmedical
center.com
www.naturalhealthmedicalcenter.
com

New Jersey's Family Holistic
Health & Acupuncture Center
206 Broad St.
Red Bank, NJ 07701
(732) 219-1900
info@NJHolistic.net
www.njholistic.net

New Seasons Natural Medicine
5 Oak Hill Rd.
Harvard, MA 01451
(978) 456-7789
Fax: (978) 456-7790
Janet@JanetBeaty.com
www.janetbeaty.com

New York ME/CFS Center
860 Fifth Ave., Suite 1C
New York, NY 10065
(212) 794-2000
Fax: (212) 327-2125
www.enlander.com

North Coast Family Health
500 Market St., Suite 1F
Portsmouth, NH 03801
(603) 427-6800
Fax: (603) 427-2801
info@naturopathic-doctors.com
www.naturopathic-doctors.com

Northampton Wellness Associates
395 Pleasant St.
Northampton, MA 01060
(413) 584-7787
Fax: (413) 584-7778
www.northamptonwellness.com

Perlmutter Health Center
800 Goodlette Rd. N, Suite 270
Naples, FL 34102
(239) 649-7400
Fax: (239) 649-6370
newpatient@perlhealth.com
www.perlhealth.com

Plymouth Integrative Medicine
Center
36650 Five Mile Rd., Suite 100
Livonia, MI 48154
(734) 432-1900
info@doctormetro.com
www.doctormetro.com

Rothfeld Center & Apothecary
411 Waverley Oaks Rd., Building
3, Suite 319
Waltham, MA 02452
(781) 736-1901
Fax: (781) 736-1911
info@rothfeldcenter.com
wholehealthne.com

Tahoma Clinic
6839 Fort Dent Way, #134
Tukwila, WA 98188
(206) 812-9988
Fax: (206) 812-9989
www.tahomaclinic.com

Tracy Darling, MD
Integrative Nutritional Medicine
31639 South Coast Hwy.
Laguna Beach, CA 92651
(949) 610-9950
Fax: (949) 612-6392

doc@darlingmd.com
www.darlingmd.com

Treatment Center for Chronic Fatigue Syndrome (CFS)
A. Martin Lerner, MD, MACP
32804 Pierce Rd.
Beverly Hills, MI 48025
(248) 540-9866
Fax: (248) 540-0139
drlerner@treatmentcenter
forcfs.com
www.treatmentcenterforcfs.com

UCSF Medical Center
500 Parnassus Ave.
San Francisco, CA 94143
(415) 476-1000
www.ucsfhealth.org

University of Maryland Medical
Center (UMMC)
22 S Greene St.
Baltimore, MD 21201
(410) 328-1500
webmaster@umms.org
www.umm.edu

University of Oklahoma College
of Medicine
Department of Neurology
1100 N Lindsay Ave.
Oklahoma City, OK 73104
(405) 271-4000
www.oumedicine.com

University of Pittsburgh Medical
Center (UPMC)

200 Lothrop St.
Pittsburgh, PA 15213
(412) 647-2345
www.upmc.edu

The Wellness Pros
471 Division St.
Campbell, CA 95008
(408) 871-8222
wellnesspros1@gmail.com
www.brainbasedcare.com

Whole Health Chicago
2522 North Lincoln Ave.
Chicago, IL 60614
(773) 296-6700
Fax: (773) 296-1131
www.wholehealthchicago.com

Winchester Natural Health Associates
10 Converse Place
Winchester, MA 01890
(781) 721-4585
Fax: (781) 569-0405
wnha@winchesternaturalhealth
.com
www.winchesternaturalhealth
.com

Woodlands Medical Center
5724 Clymer Rd.
Quakertown, PA 18951
(215) 536-1890
Fax: (215) 529-9034
www.woodmed.com

APPENDIX E

For Further Reading

Bell, David S. *The Doctor's Guide to Chronic Fatigue Syndrome: Understanding, Treating, and Living with CFIDS*. Boston: Da Capo Press, 1995.

Bested, Alison, Russell Howe, and Alan Logan. *Hope and Help for Chronic Fatigue Syndrome and Fibromyalgia*. Nashville, TN: Cumberland House, 2008.

Campling, Frankie, and Michael Sharpe. *Chronic Fatigue Syndrome*. 2nd ed. New York: Oxford University Press, 2008.

Colbert, Don. *The New Bible Cure for Chronic Fatigue & Fibromyalgia: Ancient Truths, Natural Remedies, and the Latest Findings for Your Health Today*. Lake Mary, FL: Charisma House, 2011.

Cooper, Celeste, and Jeffrey Miller. *Integrative Therapies for Fibromyalgia, Chronic Fatigue Syndrome, and Myofascial Pain: The Mind-Body Connection*. Rochester, VT: Inner Traditions International, 2010.

Cox, Diane. *Occupational Therapy and Chronic Fatigue Syndrome*. Hoboken, NJ: John Wiley & Sons, 2000.

Craggs-Hinton, Christine. *How to Manage Chronic Fatigue*. New York: Perseus Book Group, 2012.

Dantini, Daniel C. *The New Fibromyalgia Remedy: Stop Your Pain Now with an Anti-Viral Regimen*. Omaha, NE: Addicus Books, 2008.

Engdahl, Sylvia. *Chronic Fatigue Syndrome*. Farmington Hills, MI: Greenhaven Press, 2012.

Englebienne, Patrick, and Kenny De Meirleir. *Chronic Fatigue Syndrome: A Biological Approach*. Boca Raton, FL: CRC Press, 2002.

Friedberg, Fred. *Coping with Chronic Fatigue Syndrome: Nine Things You Can Do*. Oakland, CA: New Harbinger Publications, 1995.

Jason, Leonard A., Patricia A. Fennell, and Renée R. Taylor. *Handbook of Chronic Fatigue Syndrome*. Hoboken, NJ: John Wiley & Sons, 2003.

Kenny, Timothy, and Paul R. Cheney. *Living with Chronic Fatigue Syndrome: A Personal Story of the Struggle for Recovery*. New York: Thunder's Mouth Press, 1994.

Montero, Roberto Patarca. *Chronic Fatigue Syndrome and the Body's Immune Defense System: What Does the Research Say?* Boca Raton, FL: CRC Press, 2002.

Montero, Roberto Patarca, and Kenny De Meirleir. *Chronic Fatigue Syndrome: Critical Reviews and Clinical Advances—What Does the Research Say?* Boca Raton, FL: CRC Press, 2000.

Murphree, Rodger H. *Treating and Beating Fibromyalgia and Chronic Fatigue Syndrome: A Step-by-Step Program Proven to Help You Get Well Again.* New York: Harrison & Hampton Publishing, 2008.

Pall, Martin. *Explaining Unexplained Illnesses: Disease Paradigm for Chronic Fatigue Syndrome, Multiple Chemical Sensitivity, Fibromyalgia, Post-Traumatic Stress Disorder, Gulf War Syndrome and Others.* Boca Raton, FL: CRC Press, 2007.

Perrin, Raymond. *The Perrin Technique: How to Beat Chronic Fatigue Syndrome/ME.* New York: Perseus Book Group, 2007.

Shlomo, Yehuda, and David I. Mostofsky. *Chronic Fatigue Syndrome.* New York: Plenum Press, 1997.

Shomon, Mary J. *Living Well with Chronic Fatigue Syndrome and Fibromyalgia: What Your Doctor Doesn't Tell You . . . That You Need to Know.* New York: Harper Collins Publishers, 2004.

Skloot, Floyd . *The Night-Side: Chronic Fatigue Syndrome & the Illness Experience.* Brownsville, OR: Story Line, 1996.

Stoff, Jesse A. *Chronic Fatigue Syndrome.* New York: Harper Perennial, 1992.

Taylor, Renee R. *Cognitive Behavioral Therapy for Chronic Illness and Disability.* New York: Springer, 2006.

Toenjes, Annette. *Musician, Heal Thyself! An Alternative Approach to Conquering Chronic Fatigue Syndrome.* Mustang, OK: Tate Publishing, 2014.

Wessely, Simon, Matthew Hotopf, and Michael Sharpe. *Chronic Fatigue and Its Syndromes.* New York: Oxford University Press, 1999.

NOTES

PREFACE

1. "Chronic Fatigue Syndrome," accessed May 17, 2014, www.nhs.uk/conditions/Chronic-fatigue-syndrome/Pages/Introduction.aspx; "Chronic Fatigue Syndrome," accessed May 17, 2014, www.cdc.gov/cfs.

2. "Chronic Fatigue Syndrome," accessed May 17, 2014, www.patient.co.uk/doctor/chronic-fatigue-syndrome.

3. "Chronic Fatigue Syndrome," accessed May 17, 2014, www.cdc.gov/cfs; "Chronic Fatigue Syndrome," accessed May 17, 2014, www.mayoclinic.org/diseases-conditions/chronic-fatigue-syndrome/basics/definition/con-20022009.

4. "Chronic Fatigue Syndrome," accessed May 17, 2014, www.mayoclinic.org/diseases-conditions/chronic-fatigue-syndrome/basics/definition/con-20022009.

5. "Chronic Fatigue Syndrome," accessed May 17, 2014, www.patient.co.uk/doctor/chronic-fatigue-syndrome.

6. "Chronic Fatigue Syndrome," accessed May 17, 2014, www.patient.co.uk/doctor/chronic-fatigue-syndrome.

7. "Chronic Fatigue Syndrome," accessed May 17, 2014, www.cdc.gov/cfs.

8. "Chronic Fatigue Syndrome," accessed May 17, 2014, www.patient.co.uk/doctor/chronic-fatigue-syndrome.

9. "Chronic Fatigue Syndrome," accessed May 17, 2014, www.patient.co.uk/doctor/chronic-fatigue-syndrome.

10. "Chronic Fatigue Syndrome," accessed May 17, 2014, www.cdc.gov/cfs.

11. "Chronic Fatigue Syndrome," accessed May 17, 2014, www.mayoclinic.org/diseases-conditions/chronic-fatigue-syndrome/basics/definition/con-20022009; "Chronic Fatigue Syndrome," accessed May 17, 2014,

www.nhs.uk/conditions/Chronic-fatigue-syndrome/Pages/Introduction.aspx; "Chronic Fatigue Syndrome," accessed May 17, 2014, www.cdc.gov/cfs.

12. "Chronic Fatigue Syndrome," accessed May 17, 2014, www.cdc.gov/cfs; "Chronic Fatigue Syndrome," accessed May 17, 2014, www.mayoclinic.org/diseases-conditions/chronic-fatigue-syndrome/basics/definition/con-20022009; "Chronic Fatigue Syndrome," accessed May 17, 2014, www.patient.co.uk/doctor/chronic-fatigue-syndrome.

13. "Chronic Fatigue Syndrome," accessed May 17, 2014, www.patient.co.uk/doctor/chronic-fatigue-syndrome.

14. "Chronic Fatigue Syndrome," accessed May 17, 2014, www.cdc.gov/cfs; "Chronic Fatigue Syndrome," accessed May 17, 2014, www.nlm.nih.gov/medlineplus/chronicfatiguesyndrome.html.

15. "Chronic Fatigue Syndrome," accessed May 17, 2014, www.cdc.gov/cfs.

16. "Chronic Fatigue Syndrome," accessed May 17, 2014, www.cdc.gov/cfs; "Chronic Fatigue Syndrome," accessed May 17, 2014, www.patient.co.uk/doctor/chronic-fatigue-syndrome.

17. "Chronic Fatigue Syndrome," accessed May 17, 2014, www.mayoclinic.org/diseases-conditions/chronic-fatigue-syndrome/basics/definition/con-20022009.

18. "Chronic Fatigue Syndrome," accessed May 17, 2014, www.mayoclinic.org/diseases-conditions/chronic-fatigue-syndrome/basics/definition/con-20022009.

19. "Chronic Fatigue Syndrome," accessed May 17, 2014, www.mayoclinic.org/diseases-conditions/chronic-fatigue-syndrome/basics/definition/con-20022009.

20. "Chronic Fatigue Syndrome," accessed May 17, 2014, www.nhs.uk/conditions/Chronic-fatigue-syndrome/Pages/Introduction.aspx.

21. D. Dorland, *Dorland's Illustrated Medical Dictionary*, 32nd ed. (New York: Elsevier Saunders), 167.

22. "Disease—Definition," accessed May 30, 2014, www.biology-online.org/dictionary/Disease.

23. "Chronic Fatigue Syndrome," accessed May 17, 2014, www.nhs.uk/conditions/Chronic-fatigue-syndrome/Pages/Introduction.aspx; "Chronic Fatigue Syndrome," accessed May 17, 2014, www.mayoclinic.org/diseases-conditions/chronic-fatigue-syndrome/basics/definition/con-20022009.

1. ENERGY AND THE HUMAN BODY

1. J. Stedman, *Stedman's Medical Dictionary for the Health Professions and Nursing* (Baltimore: Lippincott Williams & Wilkins, 2005), 478.

2. National Sleep Foundation, "White Paper: Consequences of Drowsy Driving," accessed July 31, 2014, www.sleepfoundation.org.

3. H. Hildebrandt, M. Nübling, and V. Candia, "Increment of Fatigue, Depression, and Stage Fright during the First Year of High-level Education in Music Students," *Medical Problems of Performing Arts* 27, no. 1 (2012): 43–48.

4. G. Halvani, M. Zare, and S. Mirmohammadi, "The Relation between Shift Work, Sleepiness, Fatigue and Accidents in Iranian Industrial Mining Group Workers," *Industrial Health* 47, no. 2 (2009): 134–38.

5. B. Kozier, G. Erb, A. Berman, and S. Snyder, *Fundamentals of Nursing: Concepts, Process, and Practice* (Upper Saddle River, NJ: Pearson/Prentice Hall, 2004), 451; J. Stedman, *Stedman's Medical Dictionary for the Health Professions and Nursing* (Baltimore: Lippincott Williams & Wilkins, 2005), 1213.

6. K. Denniston, J. Topping, and R. Caret, *General, Organic, and Biochemistry* (New York: McGraw-Hill, 2007), 28.

7. B. Kozier, G. Erb, A. Berman, and S. Snyder, *Fundamentals of Nursing: Concepts, Process, and Practice* (Upper Saddle River, NJ: Pearson/Prentice Hall, 2004), 1077.

8. M. Cohen, B. Del Giorno, J. Harlan, A. McCormack, and J. Staver, *Science* (Glenview, IL: Scott Foresman & Co., 1984), 193.

9. M. Cohen, B. Del Giorno, J. Harlan, A. McCormack, and J. Staver, *Science* (Glenview, IL: Scott Foresman & Co., 1984), 6–7.

10. K. Denniston, J. Topping, and R. Caret, *General, Organic, and Biochemistry* (New York: McGraw-Hill, 2007), 28.

11. N. Campbell and J. Reece, *Essentials of Biology* (Singapore: Jurong, 2007), 1026; J. Stedman, *Stedman's Medical Dictionary for the Health Professions and Nursing* (Baltimore: Lippincott Williams & Wilkins, 2005), 155.

12. S. Smeltzer, B. Bare, J. Hinkle, and K. Cheever, *Brunner & Suddarth's Textbook of Medical-Surgical Nursing* (Baltimore: Lippincott Williams & Wilkins, 2008), 2129.

13. S. Smeltzer, B. Bare, J. Hinkle, and K. Cheever, *Brunner & Suddarth's Textbook of Medical-Surgical Nursing* (Baltimore: Lippincott Williams & Wilkins, 2008), 553.

14. L. Segers, R. Shannon, and B. Lindsey, "Interactions between Rostral Pontine and Ventral Medullary Respiratory Neurons," *Journal of Neurophysiology* 54, no. 2 (1985): 318–34.

15. N. Campbell and J. Reece, *Essentials of Biology* (Singapore: Jurong, 2007), 890.

16. S. Smeltzer, B. Bare, J. Hinkle, and K. Cheever, *Brunner & Suddarth's Textbook of Medical-Surgical Nursing* (Baltimore: Lippincott Williams & Wilkins, 2008), 2337–38.

2. HISTORY OF CHRONIC FATIGUE SYNDROME

1. L. Lorusso, S. Mikhaylova, E. Capelli, D. Ferrari, G. Ngonga, and G. Ricevuti, "Immunological Aspects of Chronic Fatigue Syndrome," *Autoimmunity Reviews* 8, no. 4 (2009): 287–91.

2. G. Holmes, J. Kaplan, N. Gantz, A. Komaroff, L. Schonberger, S. Straus, J. Jones, R. Dubois, C. Cunningham-Rundles, and S. Pahwa, "Chronic Fatigue Syndrome: A Working Case Definition," *Annals of Internal Medicine* 108, no. 3 (1988): 387– 89.

3. R. Manningham, *The Symptoms, Nature, Causes and Cure of the Februlica or Little Fever; Commonly Called the Nervous or Hysteric Fever; The Fever On The Spirits; Vapours, Hypo or Spleen* (London, 1750), 52– 53.

4. H. Deale and S. Adams, "Neurasthenia in Young Women," *American Journal of the Medical Sciences* 107, no. 4 (1894): 441.

5. G. Beard, "Neurasthenia, or Nervous Exhaustion," *The Boston Medical and Surgical Journal* (1869): 217–21.

6. H. Deale and S. Adams, "Neurasthenia in Young Women," *American Journal of the Medical Sciences* 107, no. 4 (1894): 441.

7. C. Neu, "Treatment and Management of the Neurasthenic Individual," in *Chronic Fatigue and Its Syndromes*, ed. S. Wessely, M. Hotopf, and M. Sharpe (Oxford: Oxford University Press, 1998), 106.

8. D. Young, "Florence Nightingale's Fever," *British Medical Journal* 311 (1995): 1697–1700.

9. S. Wessely, M. Hotopf, and M. Sharpe, eds., *Chronic Fatigue and Its Syndromes* (Oxford: Oxford University Press, 1998), 106.

10. D. Young, "Florence Nightingale's Fever," *British Medical Journal* 311 (1995): 1697–1700.

11. D. Young, "Florence Nightingale's Fever," *British Medical Journal* 311 (1995): 1697–1700.

12. D. Young, "Florence Nightingale's Fever," *British Medical Journal* 311 (1995): 1697–1700.

13. B. Evengard, R. Schacterle, and A. Komaroff, "Chronic Fatigue Syndrome: New Insights and Old Ignorance," *Journal of Internal Medicine* 246, no. 5 (1999): 455–69.

14. International Classification of Diseases, Tenth Revision (ICD-10) (Geneva: World Health Organization, 1992); J. Flaskerud, "Neurasthenia: Here and There, Now and Then," *Issues in Mental Health Nursing* 28, no. 6 (2007): 657–59.

15. A. MacIntyre, *M.E.: Chronic Fatigue Syndrome—A Practical Guide* (New York: Thorsons, 1998).

16. R. Patarca-Montero, *Medical Etiology, Assessment, and Treatment of Chronic Fatigue and Malaise* (Philadelphia: Haworth Press, 2004) 6–7.

17. A. Gilliam, "Epidemiological Study of an Epidemic Diagnosed as Polio-myelitis Occurring among the Personnel of the Los Angeles County General Hospital during the Summer of 1934," *Public Health Bulletin* 240 (1938).

18. R. Blattner, "Benign Myalgic Encephalomyelitis (Akureyri Disease, Ice-land Disease)," *Journal of Pediatrics* 49, no. 4 (1956): 504–6.

19. A. MacIntyre, *M.E.: Chronic Fatigue Syndrome—A Practical Guide* (New York: Thorsons, 1998).

20. B. Sigurdsson, J. Sigursonsson, J. Sigurdsson, J. Thorkelsson, and K. Gudmondsson, "A Disease Epidemic in Iceland Simulating Poliomyelitis," *American Journal of Epidemiology* (1950): 222–38.

21. S. Wessely, *Chronic Fatigue and Its Syndromes* (Oxford: Oxford University Press, 1998), 105.

22. J. Parish, "Early Outbreaks of 'Epidemic Neuromyasthenia,'" *Postgraduate Medical Journal* 54, no. 637 (1978): 711–17.

23. J. Parish, "Early Outbreaks of 'Epidemic Neuromyasthenia,'" *Postgraduate Medical Journal* 54, no. 637 (1978): 711–17.

24. M. Ramsay, "Myalgic Encephalomyelitis: A Baffling Syndrome with a Tragic Aftermath," accessed June 24, 2014, www.meactionuk.org.uk/ramsey.html.

25. M. Ramsay, "Myalgic Encephalomyelitis: A Baffling Syndrome with a Tragic Aftermath," accessed June 24, 2014, www.meactionuk.org.uk/ramsey.html.

26. C. Shepherd, *Living with M.E.* (London: Vermillion, 1999), 21.

27. P. Levine, P. Snow, B. Ranum, C. Paul, and M. Holmes, "Epidemic Neuromyasthenia and Chronic Fatigue Syndrome in West Otago, New Zea-land: A 10-year Follow-up," *Archives of Internal Medicine* 157, no. 7 (1997): 750–54.

28. N. Hashimoto, "History of Chronic Fatigue Syndrome [Article in Japa-nese]," *Nihon Rinsho* 65, no. 6 (2007): 975–82.

29. N. Hashimoto, "History of Chronic Fatigue Syndrome [Article in Japa-nese]," *Nihon Rinsho* 65, no. 6 (2007): 975–82.

30. N. Hashimoto, "History of Chronic Fatigue Syndrome [Article in Japa-nese]," *Nihon Rinsho* 65, no. 6 (2007): 975–82.

31. W. Day, "Raggedy Ann Syndrome," *Hippocrates* July/August (1987).

32. C. Mulrow, G. Ramirez, J. Cornell, and K. Allsup, "Defining and Man-aging Chronic Fatigue Syndrome: Summary," in *AHRQ Evidence Report Summaries* (Rockville, MD: Agency for Healthcare Research and Quality, 1998–2005).

33. P. Levine, J. Dale, E. Benson-Grigg, S. Fritz, S. Grufferman, and S. Straus, "A Cluster of Cases of Chronic Fatigue and Chronic Fatigue Syndrome: Clinical and Immunologic Studies," *Clinical Infectious Diseases* 23, no. 2 (1996): 408– 9.

34. G. Holmes, J. Kaplan, N. Gantz, A. Komaroff, L. Schonberger, S. Straus, J. Jones, R. Dubois, C. Cunningham-Rundles, and S. Pahwa, "Chronic Fatigue Syndrome: A Working Case Definition," *Annals of Internal Medicine* 108, no. 3 (1988): 387 – 89.

35. Tim Field Foundation, "Bullying, Stress and the Effects of Stress on Health: The Injury to Health Caused by Prolonged Negative Stress Including Fatigue, Anxiety, Depression, Immune System Suppression, IBS, Aches, Pains, Numbness and Panic Attacks," accessed August 21, 2014, www.bullyonline.org/stress/health.htm.

36. J. Richman and L. Jason, "Gender Biases Underlying the Social Construction of Illness States: The Case of Chronic Fatigue Syndrome," *Current Sociology* 49, no. 3 (2001): 15– 29.

37. G. Holmes, J. Kaplan, N. Gantz, A. Komaroff, L. Schonberger, S. Straus, J. Jones, R. Dubois, C. Cunningham-Rundles, and S. Pahwa, "Chronic Fatigue Syndrome: A Working Case Definition," *Annals of Internal Medicine* 108, no. 3 (1988): 387 – 89.

38. R. Taylor, F. Friedberg, and L. Jason, *A Clinician's Guide to Controversial Illnesses: Chronic Fatigue Syndrome, Fibromyalgia, and Multiple Chemical Sensitivities* (Sarasota, FL: Professional Resource Press, 2001).

39. L. Jason, R. Taylor, Z. Stepanek, and S. Plioplys, "Attitudes Regarding Chronic Fatigue Syndrome: The Importance of a Name," *Journal of Health Psychology* 6, no. 1 (2001): 61– 71; L. Jason, R. Taylor, S. Plioplys, Z. Stepanek, and J. Shlaes, "Evaluating Attributions for an Illness Based upon the Name: Chronic Fatigue Syndrome, Myalgic Encephalopathy and Florence Nightingale Disease," *American Journal of Community Psychology* 30, no. 1 (2002): 133– 48.

40. J. Jason, R. Taylor, Z. Stepanek, and S. Plioplys, "Attitudes Regarding Chronic Fatigue Syndrome: The Importance of a Name," *Journal of Health Psychology* 6, no. 1 (2001): 61– 71; L. Jason, R. Taylor, S. Plioplys, Z. Stepanek, and J. Shlaes, "Evaluating Attributions for an Illness Based upon the Name: Chronic Fatigue Syndrome, Myalgic Encephalopathy and Florence Nightingale Disease," *American Journal of Community Psychology* 30, no. 1 (2002): 133– 48.

41. L. Jason, C. Holbert, S. Torres-Harding, and R. Taylor, "Stigma and Chronic Fatigue Syndrome: Surveying a Name Change," *Journal of Disability Policy Studies* 14, no. 4 (2004): 222– 28.

42. L. Jason, C. Holbert, S. Torres-Harding, and R. Taylor, "Stigma and Chronic Fatigue Syndrome: Surveying a Name Change," *Journal of Disability Policy Studies* 14, no. 4 (2004): 222– 28.

43. L. Jason, C. Holbert, S. Torres-Harding, and R. Taylor, "Stigma and Chronic Fatigue Syndrome: Surveying a Name Change," *Journal of Disability Policy Studies* 14, no. 4 (2004): 222– 28.

44. L. Jason, C. Holbert, S. Torres-Harding, and R. Taylor, "Stigma and Chronic Fatigue Syndrome: Surveying a Name Change," *Journal of Disability Policy Studies* 14, no. 4 (2004): 222– 28.

45. L. Jason, C. Holbert, S. Torres-Harding, and R. Taylor, "Stigma and Chronic Fatigue Syndrome: Surveying a Name Change," *Journal of Disability Policy Studies* 14, no. 4 (2004): 222– 28.

46. L. Jason, J. Richman, F. Friedberg, L. Wagner, R. Taylor, and K. Jordan, "Politics, Science, and the Emergence of a New Disease: The Case of Chronic Fatigue Syndrome," *American Psychologist* 52, no. 9 (1997): 973– 83.

47. M. Akers, Standing Fast, Battles of a Champion (n.p.: JTC Sports, Inc. 1997).

48. S. Lisman and K. Dougherty, *Chronic Fatigue Syndrome for Dummies* (Indianapolis, IN: Wiley Publishing, 2007), 297– 302.

49. S. Lisman and K. Dougherty, *Chronic Fatigue Syndrome for Dummies* (Indianapolis, IN: Wiley Publishing, 2007), 297– 302.

50. S. Lisman and K. Dougherty, *Chronic Fatigue Syndrome for Dummies* (Indianapolis, IN: Wiley Publishing, 2007), 297– 302.

51. S. Lisman and K. Dougherty, *Chronic Fatigue Syndrome for Dummies* (Indianapolis, IN: Wiley Publishing, 2007), 297– 302.

52. S. Lisman and K. Dougherty, *Chronic Fatigue Syndrome for Dummies* (Indianapolis, IN: Wiley Publishing, 2007), 297– 302.

53. "Blake Edwards Biography," accessed July 29, 2014, www.thebiographychannel.co.uk.

54. "Blake Edwards Biography," accessed July 29, 2014, www.thebiographychannel.co.uk.

55. R. Shefchik, "World Short Track Speedskating Championships—Peterson Comes Home to Finish Skating Career," *St. Paul (MN) Pioneer Press* , March 31, 2006.

56. J. Weiner, "No Medals, but These Sports Have Own Gold—Short-track Speedskating Must Overcome Image Problem," *(MN) Star Tribune* , February 2, 1988.

57. B. Murphy, "On Track: Amy Peterson Has Something to Prove As She Bids for Her Fifth Olympic Games Berth," *St. Paul (MN) Pioneer Press* , December 14, 2001.

58. "100 Greatest Singers of All Time," *Rolling Stone*, accessed May 2, 2014, www.rollingstone.com./music/lists/100-greatest-singers-of-all-time-19691231/stevie-nicks-20101202.

59. M. Brown, "Stevie Nicks: A Survivor's Story," *The Daily Telegraph*, September 8, 2007, accessed June 3, 2014; M. Dennis, "Toronto Interview," CHUM Radio, May 6, 2001, accessed June 3, 2014.

60. M. Brown, "Stevie Nicks: A Survivor's Story," *The Daily Telegraph*, September 8, 2007, accessed June 3, 2014; M. Dennis, "Toronto Interview," CHUM Radio, May 6, 2001, accessed June 3, 2014.

61. D. Bell, *CFIDS: The Disease of a Thousand Names* (New York: Pollard Publications, 1991).

3. CAUSES AND RISK FACTORS

1. U.S. National Library of Medicine, "Chronic Fatigue Syndrome," accessed July 24, 2014, www.ncbi.nlm.nih.gov.

2. U.S. National Library of Medicine, "Chronic Fatigue Syndrome," accessed July 24, 2014, www.ncbi.nlm.nih.gov.

3. "Chronic Fatigue Syndrome (CFS)," CDC.gov, last updated May 14, 2012, accessed June 3, 2014, www.cdc.gov/cfs/causes.

4. H. Simon, "Chronic Fatigue Syndrome," University of Maryland Medical Center, last updated February 7, 2012, accessed June 3, 2014, www.umm.edu/health/medical/reports/articles/chronic-fatigue-syndrome.

5. H. Simon, "Chronic Fatigue Syndrome," University of Maryland Medical Center, last updated February 7, 2012, accessed June 3, 2014, www.umm.edu/health/medical/reports/articles/chronic-fatigue-syndrome.

6. H. Simon, "Chronic Fatigue Syndrome," University of Maryland Medical Center, last updated February 7, 2012, accessed June 3, 2014, www.umm.edu/health/medical/reports/articles/chronic-fatigue-syndrome.

7. "What are Cytokines?" Sino Biological Inc., accessed June 4, 2014, www.sinobiological.com/What-Is-Cytokine-Cytokine-Definition-a-5796.html.

8. R. Patarca, "Cytokines and Chronic Fatigue Syndrome," *Annals of the New York Academy of Sciences* 933 (2001): 185–200.

9. University of South Florida (USF Health), "Chronic Fatigue Syndrome: Inherited Virus Can Cause Cognitive Dysfunction and Fatigue," ScienceDaily, July 26, 2013, accessed June 5, 2014, www.sciencedaily.com/releases/2013/07/130726092427.htm.

10. University of South Florida (USF Health), "Chronic Fatigue Syndrome: Inherited Virus Can Cause Cognitive Dysfunction and Fatigue," ScienceDaily,

July 26, 2013, accessed June 5, 2014, www.sciencedaily.com/releases/2013/07/130726092427.htm.

11. L. Borish, K. Schmaling, J. DiClementi, J. Streib, J. Negri, and J. Jones, "Chronic Fatigue Syndrome: Identification of Distinct Subgroups on the Basis of Allergy and Psychologic Variables," *Journal of Allergy and Clinical Immunology* 102, no. 2 (1998): 222–30.

12. L. Borish, K. Schmaling, J. D. DiClementi, J. Streib, J. Negri, and J. F. Jones, "Chronic Fatigue Syndrome: Identification of Distinct Subgroups on the Basis of Allergy and Psychologic Variables," *Journal of Allergy and Clinical Immunology* 102, no. 2 (1998): 222–30.

13. "Causes of Chronic Fatigue Syndrome," NHS Choices, updated March 20, 2013, accessed June 6, 2014, www.nhs.uk/Conditions/Chronic-fatigue-syndrome/Pages/Causes.aspx.

14. M. Hanlon, "ME Is Possibly a Mental Illness—but That Does Not Mean That It Is Not Real," last updated on September 18, 2012, www.hanlonblog.dailymail.co.uk/2012/09/me-is-probably-a-mental-illness-after-all-but-that-does-not-mean-that-it-is-not-real.html.

15. "Chronic Fatigue Syndrome In-depth Report," accessed June 2, 2014, www.nytimes.com/health/guides/disease/chronic-fatigue-syndrome/print.html.

16. A. Cleare, J. Miell, E. Heap, S. Sookdeo, L. Young, G. Malhi, and V. O'Keane, "Hypothalamo-pituitary-adrenal Axis Dysfunction in Chronic Fatigue Syndrome, and the Effects of Low-dose Hydrocortisone Therapy," *The Journal of Clinical Endocrinology and Metabolism* 86, no. 8 (2001): 3545–54.

17. A. Cleare, J. Miell, E. Heap, S. Sookdeo, L. Young, G. Malhi, and V. O'Keane, "Hypothalamo-pituitary-adrenal Axis Dysfunction in Chronic Fatigue Syndrome, and the Effects of Low-dose Hydrocortisone Therapy," *The Journal of Clinical Endocrinology and Metabolism* 86, no. 8 (2001): 3545–54.

18. R. Rosmond, M. Dallman, and P. Björntorp, "Stress-related Cortisol Secretion in Men: Relationships with Abdominal Obesity and Endocrine, Metabolic and Hemodynamic Abnormalities," *The Journal of Clinical Endocrinology and Metabolism* 83, no. 6 (1998): 1853–59.

19. A. McGrady, P. Conran, D. Dickey, D. Garman, E. Farris, and C. Schumann-Brzezinski, "The Effects of Biofeedback-assisted Relaxation on Cell-mediated Immunity, Cortisol, and White Blood Cell Count in Healthy Adult Subjects," *Journal of Behavioral Medicine* 15, no. 4 (1992): 343–54.

20. H. Simon, "Chronic Fatigue Syndrome," University of Maryland Medical Center, last updated February 7, 2012, accessed June 3, 2014, www.umm.edu/health/medical/reports/articles/chronic-fatigue-syndrome.

21. "Chronic Fatigue Syndrome In-depth Report," accessed June 2, 2014, www.nytimes.com/health/guides/disease/chronic-fatigue-syndrome/print.html.

22. Mayo Clinic Staff, "Chronic Fatigue Syndrome Risk Factors," updated July 1, 2014, accessed July 5, 2014, www.mayoclinic.org/diseases-conditions/chronic-fatigue-syndrome/basics/risk-factors/con-20022009.

23. H. Simon, "Chronic Fatigue Syndrome," University of Maryland Medical Center, last updated February 7, 2012, accessed June 5, 2014, www.umm.edu/health/medical/reports/articles/chronic-fatigue-syndrome.

24. J. Issa, "The Personality of Chronic Fatigue," last updated October 22, 2010, accessed July 5, 2014, www.brainblogger.com/2010/10/22/the-personality-of-chronic-fatigue.

25. J. Issa, "The Personality of Chronic Fatigue," last updated October 22, 2010, accessed July 5, 2014, www.brainblogger.com/2010/10/22/the-personality-of-chronic-fatigue.

26. D. Ciccone, K. Busichio, M. Vickroy, and B. Natelson, "Psychiatric Morbidity in the Chronic Fatigue Syndrome: Are Patients with Personality Disorder More Physically Impaired?" *Journal of Psychosomatic Research* 54, no. 5 (2003): 445–52.

4. PATHOLOGY OF CHRONIC FATIGUE SYNDROME

1. K. Brurberg, M. Fonhus, L. Larun, S. Flottorp, and K. Malterud, "Case Definitions for Chronic Fatigue Syndrome/Myalgic Encephalomyelitis (CFS/ME): A Systematic Review," *BMJ Open* 4, no. 2 (2014): e003973.

2. E. Newsholme, E. Blomstrand, and B. Ekblom, "Physical and Mental Fatigue: Metabolic Mechanisms and Importance of Plasma Amino Acids," *British Medical Bulletin* 48, no. 3 (1992): 477–95.

3. Centers for Disease Control and Prevention, "Chronic Fatigue Syndrome: Diagnostic Tests to Exclude Other Causes," accessed May 13, 2014, www.cdc.gov/cfs/diagnosis/testing.html.

4. C. Ferri, *Chronic Fatigue Syndrome* (Quick Reference) (Chicago: Mosby, 2014), 10–12.

5. "Chronic Fatigue Syndrome/Myalgic Encephalomyelitis (or Encephalopathy) Diagnosis and Management," NICE Clinical Guideline (2007), accessed July 24, 2014, www.nice.org.uk.

6. A. Dellwo, "Chronic Fatigue Syndrome Basics Series #2," accessed May 3, 2014, www.about.com.

7. P. Plum, *Diagnosis of Stupor and Coma* (London: Oxford University Press, 2007), 5–6; Centers for Disease Control and Prevention, "Chronic Fatigue Syndrome (CFS): Symptoms," last updated May 5, 2012, accessed May 12, 2014, www.cdc.gov/cfs/symptoms/index.html.

8. L. Martínez-Martínez, T. Mora, A. Vargas, M. Fuentes-Iniestra, and M. Martínez-Lavín, "Sympathetic Nervous System Dysfunction in Fibromyalgia, Chronic Fatigue Syndrome, Irritable Bowel Syndrome, and Interstitial Cystitis: A Review of Case-control Studies," *Journal of Clinical Rheumatology* 20, no. 3 (2014): 146–50.

9. V. Giebels, H. Repping-Wuts, G. Bleijenberg, J. Kroese, N. Stikkelbroeck, and A. Hermus, "Severe Fatigue in Patients with Adrenal Insufficiency: Physical, Psychosocial and Endocrine Determinants," *Journal of Endocrinological Investigation* 37, no. 3 (2014): 293–301.

10. T. Hampton, "Researchers Find Genetic Clues to Chronic Fatigue Syndrome," *Journal of the American Medical Association* 295, no. 21 (2006): 2466–67.

11. T. Hampton, "Researchers Find Genetic Clues to Chronic Fatigue Syndrome," *Journal of the American Medical Association* 295, no. 21 (2006): 2466–67.

12. A. Pinching, "AIDS and CFS/ME: A Tale of Two Syndromes," *Clinical Medicine* 3, no. 1 (2003): 78–82.

13. E. Fuller-Thomson, R. Mehta, and J. Sulman, "Long-term Parental Unemployment in Childhood and Subsequent Chronic Fatigue Syndrome," *International Scholarly Research Notices: Family Medicine* (2013): 978250.

14. B. Natelson, M. Haghighi, and N. Ponzio, "Evidence for the Presence of Immune Dysfunction in Chronic Fatigue Syndrome," *Clinical and Diagnostic Laboratory Immunology* 9, no. 4 (2002): 747–52.

15. E. Acheson, "The Clinical Syndrome Variously Called Benign Myalgic Encephalomyelitis," *American Journal of Medicine* 26, no. 4 (1959): 569–95.

16. C. Davis, "Chronic Fatigue Syndrome: Symptoms," 2013, accessed June 23, 2014, www.medicinenet.com.

17. E. Acheson, "The Clinical Syndrome Variously Called Benign Myalgic Encephalomyelitis," *American Journal of Medicine* 26, no. 4 (1959): 569–95.

18. R. Moss-Morris V. Deary, and B. Castell, "Chronic Fatigue Syndrome," *Handbook of Clinical Neurology* 110 (2013): 303–14.

19. R. Moss-Morris, V. Deary, and B. Castell, "Chronic Fatigue Syndrome," *Handbook of Clinical Neurology* 110 (2013): 303–14.

20. R. Kilden, "Chronic Fatigue Syndrome: The Male Disorder That Became a Female Disorder," Science Daily, 2014, accessed August 2, 2014, www.Sciencedaily.com.

21. C. Davis, "Chronic Fatigue Syndrome: Symptoms," 2013, accessed June 23, 2014, www.medicinenet.com.

22. E. Gleichgerrcht and J. Decety, "The Relationship between Different Facets of Empathy, Pain Perception and Compassion Fatigue among Physicians," *Frontiers in Behavioral Neuroscience* 8 (2014): 243.

23. S. Love, *Menopause & Hormone Book: Making Informed Choices* (New York: Harmony, 2003), 103.

24. S. Love, *Menopause & Hormone Book: Making Informed Choices* (New York: Harmony, 2003), 103.

25. E. Crawley, "The Epidemiology of Chronic Fatigue Syndrome/Myalgic Encephalitis in Children," *Archives of Disease in Childhood* 99, no. 2 (2014): 171–74.

26. E. Crawley, "The Epidemiology of Chronic Fatigue Syndrome/Myalgic Encephalitis in Children," *Archives of Disease in Childhood* 99, no. 2 (2014): 171–74.

27. D. Barron, B. Cohen, M. Geraghty, R. Violand, and P. Rowe, "Joint Hypermobility Is More Common in Children with Chronic Fatigue Syndrome Than in Healthy Controls," *Journal of Pediatrics* 141, no. 3 (2002): 421.

28. D. Barron, B. Cohen, M. Geraghty, R. Violand, and P. Rowe, "Joint Hypermobility Is More Common in Children with Chronic Fatigue Syndrome Than in Healthy Controls," *Journal of Pediatrics* 141, no. 3 (2002): 421.

29. T. Chalder, J. Tong, and V. Deary, "Family Cognitive Behaviour Therapy for Chronic Fatigue Syndrome: An Uncontrolled Study," *Archives of Disease in Childhood* 86, no. 2 (2002): 95–97.

30. D. Cook, "Functional Neuroimaging Correlates of Mental Fatigue Induced by Cognition among Chronic Fatigue Syndrome Patients and Controls," *NeuroImage* 36, no. 1 (2007): 108–22.

31. D. Cook, "Functional Neuroimaging Correlates of Mental Fatigue Induced by Cognition among Chronic Fatigue Syndrome Patients and Controls," *NeuroImage* 36, no. 1 (2007): 108–22.

32. K. Miwa and M. Fujita, "Electrocardiographic QT Interval and Cardiovascular Reactivity in Fibromyalgia Differ from Chronic Fatigue Syndrome," *Clinical Cardiology* 19, no. 3 (2011): 782–86.

33. K. Rahman, A. Burton, S. Galbraith, A. Lloyd, and U. Vollmer-Conna, "Sleep-wake Behavior in Chronic Fatigue Syndrome," *Sleep* 34, no. 5 (2011): 671–78.

34. K. Rahman, A. Burton, S. Galbraith, A. Lloyd, and U. Vollmer-Conna, "Sleep-wake Behavior in Chronic Fatigue Syndrome," *Sleep* 34, no. 5 (2011): 671–78.

35. K. Rahman, A. Burton, S. Galbraith, A. Lloyd, and U. Vollmer-Conna, "Sleep-wake Behavior in Chronic Fatigue Syndrome," Sleep 34, no. 5 (2011): 671–78.

36. J. Naschitz, M. Fields, H. Isseroff, D. Sharif, E. Sabo, and I. Rosner, "Shortened QT Interval: A Distinctive Feature of the Dysautonomia of Chronic Fatigue Syndrome," *Journal of Electrocardiology* 39, no. 4 (2006): 389–94.

37. J. Naschitz, M. Fields, H. Isseroff, D. Sharif, E. Sabo, and I. Rosner, "Shortened QT Interval: A Distinctive Feature of the Dysautonomia of Chronic Fatigue Syndrome," *Journal of Electrocardiology* 39, no. 4 (2006): 389–94.

38. R. Antiel, J. Caudill, B. Burkhardt, C. Brands, and P. Fischer, "Iron, Insufficiency and Hypovitaminosis D in Adolescents with Chronic Fatigue and Orthostatic Intolerance," *Southern Medical Journal* 104, no.8 (2011): 609–11.

39. A. Hoeck, *Vitamin D Deficiency Results in Chronic Fatigue and Multisystem Symptoms* (Cologne, Germany: International Association for Chronic Fatigue Syndrome/Myalgic Encaphalomyelitis, 2009), 1–6.

40. A. Hoeck, *Vitamin D Deficiency Results in Chronic Fatigue and Multisystem Symptoms* (Cologne, Germany: International Association for Chronic Fatigue Syndrome/Myalgic Encaphalomyelitis, 2009), 1–6.

41. B. Hurwitz, V. Coryell, M. Parker, P. Martin, A. Laperriere, N. Klimas, G. Sfakianakis, and M. Bilsker, "Chronic Fatigue Syndrome: Illness Severity, Sedentary Lifestyle, Blood Volume and Evidence of Diminished Cardiac Function," *Clinical Science* 118, no. 2 (2009): 125–35.

42. B. Hurwitz, V. Coryell, M. Parker, P. Martin, A. Laperriere, N. Klimas, G. Sfakianakis, and M. Bilsker, "Chronic Fatigue Syndrome: Illness Severity, Sedentary Lifestyle, Blood Volume and Evidence of Diminished Cardiac Function," *Clinical Science* 118, no. 2 (2009): 125–35.

43. A. Lerner, "Prevalence of Abnormal Cardiac Wall Motion in the Cardiomyopathy Associated with Incomplete Multiplication of Epstein-Barr Virus and/or Cytomegalovirus in Patients with Chronic Fatigue Syndrome," *In Vivo* 18, no. 4 (2004): 417–24.

44. Centers for Disease Control and Prevention, "Chronic Fatigue Syndrome (CFS), Symptoms," last updated May 5, 2012, accessed June 2, 2014, www.cdc.gov/cfs/symptoms/index.html.

45. T. Muayqil, G. Gronseth, and R. Camicioli, "Evidence-based Guideline: Diagnostic Accuracy of CSF 14-3-3 Protein in Sporadic Creutzfeldt-Jakob Disease: Report of the Guideline Development Subcommittee of the American Academy of Neurology," *Neurology* 79, no. 14 (2012): 1499–506.

46. E. Verrillo, *Chronic Fatigue Syndrome: A Treatment Guide*, 2nd ed. (Seattle, WA: Erica Verrillo, 2012).

5. DIAGNOSING CHRONIC FATIGUE SYNDROME

1. M. Sharpe, L. Archard, J. Banatvala, L. Borysiewicz, A. Clare, A. David, R. Edwards, K. Hawton, H. Lambert, R. Lane, E. McDonald, J. Mowbray, D. Pearson, T. Peto, V. Preedy, A. Smith, D. Smith, D. Taylor, D. Tyrrell, S.

Wessely, and P. White, "A Report: Chronic Fatigue Syndrome: Guidelines for Research," *Journal of the Royal Society of Medicine* 84, no. 2 (1991): 118–21.

2. M. Sharpe, L. Archard, J. Banatvala, L. Borysiewicz, A. Clare, A. David, R. Edwards, K. Hawton, H. Lambert, R. Lane, E. McDonald, J. Mowbray, D. Pearson, T. Peto, V. Preedy, A. Smith, D. Smith, D. Taylor, D. Tyrrell, S. Wessely, and P. White, "A Report: Chronic Fatigue Syndrome: Guidelines for Research," *Journal of the Royal Society of Medicine* 84, no. 2 (1991): 118–21.

3. E. Lattie, M. Antoni, M. Fletcher, S. Czaja, D. Perdomo, A. Sala, S. Nair, S. Hua Fu, F. Penedo, and N. Klimas, "Beyond Myalgic Encephalomye-litis/Chronic Fatigue Syndrome (ME/CFS) Symptom Severity: Stress Management Skills Are Related to Lower Illness Burden," *Fatigue* 1, no. 4 (2013): 210–22.

4. D. Bates, D. Buchwald, J. Lee, P. Kith, T. Doolittle, C. Rutherford, W. Churchill, P. Schur, M. Wener, and D. Wybenga, "Clinical Laboratory Test Findings in Patients with Chronic Fatigue Syndrome," *Archives of Internal Medicine* 155, no. 1 (1995): 97–103.

5. C. Shepherd, *Diagnosis: Delay Harms Health—Early Diagnosis: Why Is It So Important?* (London: ME Alliance, 2005), 11.

6. M. Sharpe, L. Archard, J. Banatvala, L. Borysiewicz, A. Clare, A. David, R. Edwards, K. Hawton, H. Lambert, R. Lane, E. McDonald, J. Mowbray, D. Pearson, T. Peto, V. Preedy, A. Smith, D. Smith, D. Taylor, D. Tyrrell, S. Wessely, and P. White, "A Report: Chronic Fatigue Syndrome: Guidelines for Research," *Journal of the Royal Society of Medicine* 84, no. 2 (1991): 118–21.

7. C. Shepherd, *Living with M.E.: The Chronic/Post-viral Fatigue Syndrome*, 3rd ed. (London: Random House UK, 1999).

8. G. Norman and K. Eva, "Diagnostic Error and Clinical Reasoning," *Medical Education* 44, no. 1 (2010): 94–100.

9. J. Valdizán Usón and I. Alecha, "Diagnostic and Treatment Challenges of Chronic Fatigue Syndrome: Role of Immediate-release Methylphenidate," *Expert Review of Neurotherapeutics* 8, no. 6 (2008): 917–27.

10. C. Shepherd, *Living with M.E.: The Chronic/Post-viral Fatigue Syndrome*, 3rd ed. (London: Random House UK, 1999).

11. S. Shor, "Lyme Disease Presenting As Chronic Fatigue Syndrome," *Journal of Chronic Fatigue Syndrome*, 13, no. 4 (2006).

12. S. Shor, "Lyme Disease Presenting As Chronic Fatigue Syndrome," *Journal of Chronic Fatigue Syndrome*, 13, no. 4 (2006).

13. C. Shepherd, *Living with M.E.: The Chronic/Post-viral Fatigue Syndrome*, 3rd ed. (London: Random House UK, 1999).

14. C. Ray, S. Jefferies, and W. Weir, "Life Events and the Course of Chronic Fatigue Syndrome," *British Journal of Medical Psychology*, 68, no. 4 (1995): 323–31.

15. P. White, J. Thomas, H. Kangro, W. Bruce-Jones, J. Amess, D. Craw-ford, S. Grover, and A. Clare, "Predictions and Associations of Fatigue Syndromes and Mood Disorders That Occur after Infectious Mononucleosis," *Lancet* 358, no. 9297 (2001): 1946–54.

16. A. House and H. Andrews, "Life Events and Difficulties Preceding the Onset of Functional Dysphonia," *Journal of Psychosomatic Research* 32, no. 3 (1988): 311–19; H. Andrews and A House, "Functional Dysphonia: Establishing a New Dimension of Life Events and Difficulties," in *Life Events and Illness*, ed. G. Brown and T. Harris (London: Guilford Press, 1989), 343–53.

17. C. Werker, S. Nijhof, and E. Van de Putte, "Clinical Practice: Chronic Fatigue Syndrome," *European Journal of Pediatrics* 172, no. 10 (2013): 1293–98.

18. M. Huibers, I. Kant, J. Knottnerus, G. Bleijenberg, G. Swaen, and S. Kasl, "Development of the Chronic Fatigue Syndrome in Severely Fatigued Employees: Predictors of Outcome in the Maastricht Cohort Study," *Journal of Epidemiology & Community Health* 58, no. 10 (2004): 877–82.

19. D. Buchwald and D. Garrity, "Comparison of Patients with Chronic Fatigue Syndrome, Fibromyalgia, and Multiple Chemical Sensitivities," *Archives of Internal Medicine* 154, no. 18 (1994): 2049–53.

20. D. Buchwald and D. Garrity, "Comparison of Patients with Chronic Fatigue Syndrome, Fibromyalgia, and Multiple Chemical Sensitivities," *Archives of Internal Medicine* 154, no. 18 (1994): 2049–53.

21. R. Dietert and J. Dietert, "Possible Role for Early-life Immune Insult Including Developmental Immunotoxicity in Chronic Fatigue Syndrome (CFS) or Myalgic Encephalomyelitis (ME)," *Toxicology* 247, no. 1 (2008).

22. J. Fenaux, R. Gogal Jr, and S. Ahmed, "Diethylstilbesterol Exposure during Fetal Development Affects Thymus: Studies in Fourteen-month-old Mice," *Journal of Reproductive Immunology* 64 nos. 1–2 (2004): 75–90.

23. R. Dietert and J. Dietert, "Possible Role for Early-life Immune Insult Including Developmental Immunotoxicity in Chronic Fatigue Syndrome (CFS) or Myalgic Encephalomyelitis (ME)," *Toxicology* 247, no. 1 (2008).

24. M. Espey, D. Thomas, K. Miranda, and D. Wink, "Focusing of Nitric Oxide Mediated Nitrosation and Oxidative Nitrosylation As a Consequence of Reaction with Superoxide," *Proceedings of the National Academy of Sciences* 99, no. 17 (2002): 11127–32.

25. M. Espey, D. Thomas, K. Miranda, and D. Wink, "Focusing of Nitric Oxide Mediated Nitrosation and Oxidative Nitrosylation As a Consequence of Reaction with Superoxide," *Proceedings of the National Academy of Sciences* 99, no. 17 (2002): 11127–32.

26. M. Caliguri, C. Murray, D. Buchwald, H. Levine, P. Cheney, D. Peterson, A. Komaroff, and J. Ritz, "Phenotypic and Functional Deficiency of Natu-

ral Killer Cells in Patients with Chronic Fatigue Syndrome," *Journal of Immunology* 130 (1987): 3306–13.

27. "Chronic Fatigue Syndrome," University of Maryland Medical Center (UMMC), accessed May 3, 2014, www.umm.edu/health/medical/altmed/condition/chronic-fatigue-syndrome.

28. C. Shepherd, *Living with M.E.: The Chronic/Post-viral Fatigue Syndrome*, 3rd ed. (London: Random House UK, 1999).

29. D. Goldenberg, R. Simms, A. Geiger, and A. Komaroff, "High Frequency of Fibromyalgia in Patients with Chronic Fatigue Seen in Primary Care Practice," *Arthritis & Rheumatology* 33, no. 3 (1990): 381–87.

30. C. Shepherd, *Living with M.E.: The Chronic/Post-viral Fatigue Syndrome*, 3rd ed. (London: Random House UK, 1999).

31. I. Hickie, B. Bennett, A. Lloyd, A. Heath, and N. Martin, "Complex Genetic and Environmental Relationships between Psychological Distress, Fatigue and Immune Functioning: A Twin Study," *Psychological Medicine* 29, no. 2 (1999): 269–77.

32. A. Farmer, J. Scourfield, N. Martin, A. Cardeno, and P. McGuffin, "Is Disabling Fatigue in Childhood Influenced by Genes?" *Psychological Medicine* 29, no. 2 (1999): 279–82.

33. A. Farmer, J. Scourfield, N. Martin, A. Cardeno, and P. McGuffin, "Is Disabling Fatigue in Childhood Influenced by Genes?" *Psychological Medicine* 29, no. 2 (1999): 279–82.

34. N. Afari and D. Buchwald, "Chronic Fatigue Syndrome: A Review," *American Journal of Psychiatry* 160 (2003): 221–36.

35. B. Natelson, J. Cohen, I. Brassloff, and H. Lee, "A Controlled Study of Brain Magnetic Resonance Imaging in Patients with Fatiguing Illnesses," *Journal of Neurological Science* 120, no. 2 (1993): 213–17.

36. R. Schwartz, B. Garada, A. Komaroff, H. Tice, M. Gleit, F. Jolesz, and B. Holman, "Detection of Intracranial Abnormalities in Patients with Chronic Fatigue Syndrome: Comparison of MR Imaging and SPECT," *American Journal of Roentgenology* 162, no. 4 (1994): 935–41.

37. D. Lewis, H. Mayberg, M. Fischer, J. Goldberg, S. Ashton, M. Graham, and D. Buchwald, "Monozygotic Twins Discordant for Chronic Fatigue Syndrome: Regional Cerebral Blood Flow SPECT," *Radiology* 219, no. 3 (2001): 766–73.

38. D. Torpy, A. Bachmann, J. Grice, S. Fitzgerald, P. Phillips, J. Whitworth, and R. Jackson, "Familial Corticosteroid-binding Globulin Deficiency Due to a Novel Null Mutation: Association with Fatigue and Relative Hypotension," *Journal of Clinical Endocrinology and Metabolism* 86, no. 8 (2001): 3692–700.

39. D. Torpy, A. Bachmann, J. Grice, S. Fitzgerald, P. Phillips, J. Whitworth, and R. Jackson, "Familial Corticosteroid-binding Globulin Deficiency Due to a Novel Null Mutation: Association with Fatigue and Relative Hypotension," *Journal of Clinical Endocrinology and Metabolism* 86, no. 8 (2001): 3692–700.

40. N. Afari and D. Buchwald, "Chronic Fatigue Syndrome: A Review," *American Journal of Psychiatry* 160, no. 2 (2003): 221–36.

41. S. Wessely, T. Chalder, S. Hirsch, P. Wallace, and D. Wright, "Psychological Symptoms, Somatic Symptoms, and Psychiatric Disorder in Chronic Fatigue and Chronic Fatigue Syndrome: A Prospective Study in the Primary Care Setting," *American Journal of Psychiatry* 153, no. 8 (1996): 1050–59.

42. I. Hickie, A. Lloyd, D. Wakefield, and G. Parker, "The Psychiatric Status of Patients with Chronic Fatigue Syndrome," *British Journal of Psychiatry* 156 (1990): 534–40.

43. N. Afari and D. Buchwald, "Chronic Fatigue Syndrome: A Review," *American Journal of Psychiatry* 160, no. 2 (2003): 221–36.

44. C. Surawy, A. Hackman, K. Hawton, and M. Sharpe, "Chronic Fatigue Syndrome: A Cognitive Approach," *Behaviour Research and Therapy* 33, no. 5 (1995): 534–44.

45. C. Whelton, I. Salit, and H. Moldofsky, "Sleep, Epstein-Barr Virus Infection, Musculoskeletal Pain, and Depressive Symptoms in Chronic Fatigue Syndrome," *Journal of Rheumatology* 19, no. 6 (1992): 939–43; R. Morris, M. Sharpe, A. Sharpley, P. Cowen, K. Hawton, and J. Morris, "Abnormalities of Sleep in Patients with Chronic Fatigue Syndrome," *British Medical Journal* 306 (1993): 1161–64.

46. O. Ortega-Hernandez and Y. Shoenfeld, "Infection, Vaccination, and Autoantibodies in Chronic Fatigue Syndrome, Cause or Coincidence?" *Annals of the New York Academy of Sciences* 1173 (2009): 600–609.

47. M. Hotopf and S. Wessely, "Viruses, Neurosis and Fatigue," *Journal of Psychosomatic Research* 38, no. 6 (1994): 499–514.

6. ROLES OF THE FAMILY PHYSICIAN, INTERNIST, AND NEUROLOGIST IN CHRONIC FATIGUE SYNDROME

1. J. Bowen, D. Pheby, A. Charlett, and C. McNulty, "Chronic Fatigue Syndrome: A Survey of GPs' Attitudes and Knowledge," *Family Practice* 22, no. 4 (2005): 389–93.

2. D. Stevens, "Chronic Fatigue," *Western Journal of Medicine* 175, no. 5 (2001): 315–19.

3. A. Mcgaha, E. Garrett, A. Jobe, P. Nalin, W. Newton, P. Pugno, and N. Kahn, "Responses to Medical Students' Frequently Asked Questions about Family Medicine," *American Family Physician* 76, no. 1 (2007): 99–106.

4. "What Does a Family Physician Do?" Virginia Commonwealth University Medical Center Department of Family Medicine and Population Health, last modified February 8, 2013, accessed May 23, 2014, www.familymedicine.vcu.edu/patient/physician.

5. "What Does a Family Physician Do?" Virginia Commonwealth University Medical Center Department of Family Medicine and Population Health, last modified February 8, 2013, accessed May 23, 2014, www.familymedicine.vcu.edu/patient/physician.

6. L. McNaughton-Filion, "The Role of a Community Family Physician from a Resident's Viewpoint," *Canadian Family Physician* 37 (1991): 1843–45.

7. A. Mcgaha, E. Garrett, A. Jobe, P. Nalin, W. Newton, P. Pugno, and N. Kahn, "Responses to Medical Students' Frequently Asked Questions about Family Medicine," *American Family Physician* 76, no. 1 (2007): 99–106.

8. D. Mueller, "Medical Student Perspectives: What Are the Differences between Internal Medicine and Family Medicine," American College of Physicians, last modified 2011, accessed June 2, 2014, www.acponline.org/medical_students/impact/archives/2010/12/perspect/.

9. D. Mueller, "Medical Student Perspectives: What Are the Differences between Internal Medicine and Family Medicine," American College of Physicians, last modified 2011, accessed June 2, 2014, www.acponline.org/medical_students/impact/archives/2010/12/perspect/.

10. D. Mueller, "Medical Student Perspectives: What Are the Differences between Internal Medicine and Family Medicine," American College of Physicians, last modified 2011, accessed June 2, 2014, www.acponline.org/medical_students/impact/archives/2010/12/perspect/.

11. D. Robinson, "The Internist's Role in Treating Fibromyalgia & Chronic Fatigue Syndrome," ProHealth, October 20, 2003, accessed June 4, 2014, www.prohealth.com/library/showarticle.cfm?libid=9927.

12. Y. Cheng-Chee, "1st College of Physicians Lecture: The Role of Internal Medicine As a Specialty in the Era of Subspecialisation," *Annals of the Academy of Medicine* 33, no. 6 (2004): 725–32.

13. D. Robinson, "The Internist's Role in Treating Fibromyalgia & Chronic Fatigue Syndrome," ProHealth, October 20, 2003, accessed June 4, 2014, www.prohealth.com/library/showarticle.cfm?libid=9927.

14. D. Mueller, "Medical Student Perspectives: What Are the Differences between Internal Medicine and Family Medicine," American College of Physicians, last modified 2011, accessed June 2, 2014, www.acponline.org/medical_students/impact/archives/2010/12/perspect/.

15. Y. Cheng-Chee, "1st College of Physicians Lecture: The Role of Internal Medicine As a Specialty in the Era of Subspecialisation," *Annals of the Academy of Medicine* 33, no. 6 (2004): 725–32.

16. S. Cohn and D. Macpherson, "Overview of the Principles of Medical Consultation and Perioperative Medicine," UpToDate, last modified June 28, 2013, accessed June 5, 2014, www.uptodate.com/contents/overview-of-the-principles-of-medical-consultation-and-perioperative-medicine.

17. S. Cohn and D. Macpherson, "Overview of the Principles of Medical Consultation and Perioperative Medicine," UpToDate, last modified June 28, 2013, accessed June 5, 2014, www.uptodate.com/contents/overview-of-the-principles-of-medical-consultation-and-perioperative-medicine.

18. W. Levinson, "Preoperative Evaluations by an Internist—Are They Worthwhile?" *Western Journal of Medicine* 141, no. 3 (1984): 395–98.

19. American Academy of Neurology and American Academy of Neurology Education & Research Foundation, "What Is Neurology," Montana Neurological Associates, accessed July 9, 2014, www.montananeurosurgery.com/What_is_Neurology.

20. American Academy of Neurology and American Academy of Neurology Education & Research Foundation, "What Is Neurology," Montana Neurological Associates, accessed July 9, 2014, www.montananeurosurgery.com/What_is_Neurology.

21. T. Sabin, "An Approach to Chronic Fatigue Syndrome in Adults," *Neurologist* 9, no. 1 (2003): 28–34.

22. American Academy of Neurology and American Academy of Neurology Education & Research Foundation, "What Is Neurology," Montana Neurological Associates, accessed July 9, 2014, http://www.montananeurosurgery.com/What_is_Neurology.

23. L. Kelchner, "The Duties of a Neurologist," accessed July 9, 2014, www.work.chron.com/duties-neurologist-12344.html.

24. L. Kelchner, "The Duties of a Neurologist," accessed July 9, 2014, www.work.chron.com/duties-neurologist-12344.html.

25. T. Sabin, "An Approach to Chronic Fatigue Syndrome in Adults," *Neurologist* 9, no. 1 (2003): 28–34.

26. L. Kelchner, "The Duties of a Neurologist," accessed July 9, 2014, www.work.chron.com/duties-neurologist-12344.html.

27. L. Kelchner, "The Duties of a Neurologist," accessed July 9, 2014, www.work.chron.com/duties-neurologist-12344.html.

28. L. Kelchner, "The Duties of a Neurologist," accessed July 9, 2014, www.work.chron.com/duties-neurologist-12344.html.

29. S. Gluckman, "Clinical Features and Diagnosis of Chronic Fatigue Syndrome," UpToDate, last modified November 26, 2013, accessed May 23, 2014,

www.uptodate.com/contents/clinical-features-and-diagnosis-of-chronic-fatigue-syndrome.

30. J. McSherry, "Chronic Fatigue Syndrome: A Fresh Look at an Old Problem, *Canadian Family Physician* 39 (1993): 336–40.

31. C. DiMaria, "CFS (Chronic Fatigue Syndrome)," Healthline, July 18, 2012, accessed May 23, 2014, www.healthline.com/health/chronic-fatigue-syndrome#Overview1.

32. F. Albright, K. Light, A. Light, L. Bateman, and L. Cannon-Albright, "Evidence for a Heritable Predisposition to Chronic Fatigue Syndrome," *BMC Neurology* 11 (2011): 62.

33. C. DiMaria, "CFS (Chronic Fatigue Syndrome)," Healthline, July 18, 2012, accessed May 23, 2014, www.healthline.com/health/chronic-fatigue-syndrome#Overview1.

34. S. Gluckman, "Patient Information: Chronic Fatigue Syndrome (Beyond the Basics)," UpToDate, last modified March 3, 2014, accessed May 23, 2014, www.uptodate.com/contents/chronic-fatigue-syndrome-beyond-the-basics.

35. S. Gluckman, "Patient Information: Chronic Fatigue Syndrome (Beyond the Basics)," UpToDate, last modified March 3, 2014, accessed May 23, 2014, www.uptodate.com/contents/chronic-fatigue-syndrome-beyond-the-basics.

36. S. Gluckman, "Patient Information: Chronic Fatigue Syndrome (Beyond the Basics)," UpToDate, last modified March 3, 2014, accessed May 23, 2014, www.uptodate.com/contents/chronic-fatigue-syndrome-beyond-the-basics.

37. A. Bested, P. Saunders, and A. Logan, "Chronic Fatigue Syndrome: Neurological Findings May Be Related to Blood-Brain Barrier Permeability," *Medical Hypotheses* 57, no. 2 (2001): 231–37.

38. Georgetown University Medical Center, "Research Provides More Evidence That Chronic Fatigue Syndrome Is a Legitimate Medical Condition," Science Daily, accessed July 9, 2014, www.sciencedaily.com/releases/2006/01/060110013424.htm.

39. Georgetown University Medical Center, "Research Provides More Evidence That Chronic Fatigue Syndrome Is a Legitimate Medical Condition," Science Daily, accessed July 9, 2014, www.sciencedaily.com/releases/2006/01/060110013424.htm.

40. A. Fernandez, A. Martin, M. Martinez, M. Bustillo, F. Hernandez, J. Labrado, R. Peñas, E. Rivas, C. Delgado, J. Redondo, and J. Gimenez, "Chronic Fatigue Syndrome: Aetiology, Diagnosis, and Treatment," *BioMed Central Psychiatry* 9, Suppl. 1 (2009): S1.

41. J. McSherry, "Chronic Fatigue Syndrome: A Fresh Look at an Old Problem," *Canadian Family Physician* 39 (1993): 336–40.

42. S. Kreijkamp-Kaspers, E. Brenu, S. Marshall, D. Staines, and M. Van Driel, "Treating Chronic Fatigue Syndrome—A Study into the Scientific Evidence for Pharmacological Treatments," *Australian Family Physician* 40, no. 11 (2011): 907–12.

43. Georgetown University Medical Center, "Research Provides More Evidence That Chronic Fatigue Syndrome Is a Legitimate Medical Condition," Science Daily, accessed July 9, 2014, www.sciencedaily.com/releases/2006/01/060110013424.htm.

44. A. Fernandez, A. Martin, M. Martinez, M. Bustillo, F. Hernandez, J. Labrado, R. Peñas, E. Rivas, C. Delgado, J. Redondo, and J. Gimenez, "Chronic Fatigue Syndrome: Aetiology, Diagnosis, and Treatment," *BioMed Central Psychiatry* 9, Suppl. 1 (2009): S1.

45. J. McSherry, "Chronic Fatigue Syndrome: A Fresh Look at an Old Problem," *Canadian Family Physician* 39 (1993): 336–40.

46. A. Fernandez, A. Martin, M. Martinez, M. Bustillo, F. Hernandez, J. Labrado, R. Peñas, E. Rivas, C. Delgado, J. Redondo, and J. Gimenez, "Chronic Fatigue Syndrome: Aetiology, Diagnosis, and Treatment," *BioMed Central Psychiatry* 9, Suppl. 1 (2009): S1.

47. A. Fernandez, A. Martin, M. Martinez, M. Bustillo, F. Hernandez, J. Labrado, R. Peñas, E. Rivas, C. Delgado, J. Redondo, and J. Gimenez, "Chronic Fatigue Syndrome: Aetiology, Diagnosis, and Treatment," *BioMed Central Psychiatry* 9, Suppl. 1 (2009): S1.

48. A. Fernandez, A. Martin, M. Martinez, M. Bustillo, F. Hernandez, J. Labrado, R. Peñas, E. Rivas, C. Delgado, J. Redondo, and J. Gimenez, "Chronic Fatigue Syndrome: Aetiology, Diagnosis, and Treatment," *BioMed Central Psychiatry* 9, Suppl. 1 (2009): S1.

49. S. Attfield, A. Adams, and A. Blandford, "Patient Information Needs: Pre- and Post-consultation," *Health Informatics Journal* 12, no. 2 (2006): 165–77.

50. C. King and L. Jason, "Improving the Diagnostic Criteria and Procedures for Chronic Fatigue Syndrome," *Biological Psychology* 68, no. 2 (2005): 87–106.

51. A. Fernandez, A. Martin, M. Martinez, M. Bustillo, F. Hernandez, J. Labrado, R. Peñas, E. Rivas, C. Delgado, J. Redondo, and J. Gimenez, "Chronic Fatigue Syndrome: Aetiology, Diagnosis, and Treatment," *BioMed Central Psychiatry* 9, Suppl. 1 (2009): S1.

52. M. Brown, A. Brown, and L. Jason, "Illness Duration and Coping Style in Chronic Fatigue Syndrome," *Psychological Reports* 106, no. 2 (2010): 383–93.

53. M. Brown, A. Brown, and L. Jason, "Illness Duration and Coping Style in Chronic Fatigue Syndrome," *Psychological Reports* 106, no. 2 (2010): 383–93.

54. L. Cordingley, A. Wearden, L. Appleby, and L. Fisher, "The Family Response Questionnaire: A New Scale to Assess the Responses of Family Members to People with Chronic Fatigue Syndrome," *Journal of Psychosomatic Research* 51, no. 2 (2001): 417–24.

55. L. Cordingley, A. Wearden, L. Appleby, and L. Fisher, "The Family Response Questionnaire: A New Scale to Assess the Responses of Family Members to People with Chronic Fatigue Syndrome," *Journal of Psychosomatic Research* 51, no. 2 (2001): 417–24.

56. "Causes of Chronic Fatigue Syndrome," NHS Choices, last modified March 20, 2013, accessed May 24, 2014, www.nhs.uk/Conditions/Chronic-fatigue-syndrome/Pages/Causes.aspx.

57. "Causes of Chronic Fatigue Syndrome," NHS Choices, last modified March 20, 2013, accessed May 24, 2014, www.nhs.uk/Conditions/Chronic-fatigue-syndrome/Pages/Causes.aspx.

58. "Causes of Chronic Fatigue Syndrome," NHS Choices, last modified March 20, 2013, accessed May 24, 2014, www.nhs.uk/Conditions/Chronic-fatigue-syndrome/Pages/Causes.aspx.

59. D. Saltman, N. O'Dea, and M. Kidd, "Conflict Management: A Primer for Doctors in Training," *Postgraduate Medical Journal* 82, no. 963 (2006): 9–12.

60. S. Gluckman, "Treatment of Chronic Fatigue Syndrome," UpToDate, last modified June 25, 2013, accessed May 24, 2014, www.uptodate.com/contents/treatment-of-chronic-fatigue-syndrome.

61. A. Helfer, A. Camargo, N. Tavares, P. Kanavos, and A. Bertoldi, "Affordability and Availability of Drugs for Treatment of Chronic Diseases in the Public Health Care System [Article in Portuguese]," *Revista Panamericana de Salud Pública* 31, no. 3 (2012): 225–32.

7. ROLE OF THE HOSPITAL IN CHRONIC FATIGUE SYNDROME

1. "Chronic Fatigue Syndrome (CFS)/Diagnosis," Centers for Disease Control and Prevention, last modified May 14, 2012, accessed July 4, 2014. www.cdc.gov/cfs/diagnosis.

2. "Chronic Fatigue Syndrome (CFS)/Diagnosis," Centers for Disease Control and Prevention, last modified May 14, 2012, accessed July 4, 2014. www.cdc.gov/cfs/diagnosis.

3. S. Gluckman, "Patient Information: Chronic Fatigue Syndrome (Beyond the Basics)," last updated March 3, 2014, accessed July 5, 2014, www.uptodate.com.

4. S. Gluckman, "Patient Information: Chronic Fatigue Syndrome (Beyond the Basics)," last updated March 3, 2014, accessed July 5, 2014, www.uptodate.com.

5. H. Aiken, P. Clarke, M. Sloane, T. Lake, and T. Cheney, "Effects of Hospital Environment on Patient Mortality and Nurse Outcome," *The Journal of Nursing Administration* 38, no. 5 (2008): 223–29.

6. H. Aiken, P. Clarke, M. Sloane, T. Lake, and T. Cheney, "Effects of Hospital Environment on Patient Mortality and Nurse Outcome," *The Journal of Nursing Administration* 38, no. 5 (2008): 223–29.

7. H. Aiken, P. Clarke, M. Sloane, T. Lake, and T. Cheney, "Effects of Hospital Environment on Patient Mortality and Nurse Outcome," *The Journal of Nursing Administration* 38, no. 5 (2008): 223–29.

8. J. Pols, "Politics of Mental Illness: Myth and Power in the Work of Thomas S. Szasz," 2005, accessed July 4, 2014, www.janpols.net/Chapter-6/5.html.

9. J. Pols, "Politics of Mental Illness: Myth and Power in the Work of Thomas S. Szasz," 2005, accessed July 4, 2014, www.janpols.net/Chapter-6/5.html.

10. A. Coulter and P. Cleary, "Patients' Experiences with Hospital Care in Five Countries," *Health Affairs* 20, no. 3 (2001): 244–52.

11. E. Jacobson, W. Keough, B. Dalton, and D. Giansiracusa, "A Comparison of Inpatient and Outpatient Experiences during an Internal Medicine Clerkship," *American Journal of Medicine* 104, no. 2 (1998): 159–62.

12. E. Jacobson, W. Keough, B. Dalton, and D. Giansiracusa, "A Comparison of Inpatient and Outpatient Experiences during an Internal Medicine Clerkship," *American Journal of Medicine* 104, no. 2 (1998): 159–62.

13. D. Cox and L. Findley, "The Management of Chronic Fatigue Syndrome in an Inpatient Setting: Presentation of an Approach and Perceived Outcome," *British Journal of Occupational Therapy* 61, no. 9 (1998): 405–9.

14. E. Jacobson, W. Keough, B. Dalton, and D. Giansiracusa, "A Comparison of Inpatient and Outpatient Experiences during an Internal Medicine Clerkship," *American Journal of Medicine* 104, no. 2 (1998): 159–62.

15. B. Kozier, G. Erb, A. Berman, and S. Snyder, *Fundamentals of Nursing: Concepts, Process, and Practice*, 7th ed. (Singapore: Pearson Education South East Asia, 2004), 91.

16. S. Gluckman, "Patient Information: Chronic Fatigue Syndrome (Beyond the Basics)," last updated March 3, 2014, accessed July 5, 2014, www.uptodate.com.

17. E. Jacobson, W. Keough, B. Dalton, and D. Giansiracusa, "A Comparison of Inpatient and Outpatient Experiences during an Internal Medicine Clerkship," *American Journal of Medicine* 104, no. 2 (1998): 159–62.

18. R. Viner, A. Gregorowski, C. Wine, M. Bladen, D. Fisher, M. Miller, and S. El Neil, "Outpatient Rehabilitative Treatment of Chronic Fatigue Syndrome (CFS/ME)," *Archives of Disease in Childhood* 89, no. 7 (2004): 615–19.

19. B. Kozier, G. Erb, A. Berman, and S. J. Snyder, *Fundamentals of Nursing: Concepts, Process, and Practice*, 7th ed. (Singapore: Pearson Education South East Asia, 2004), 91.

20. R. Viner, A. Gregorowski, C. Wine, M. Bladen, D. Fisher, M. Miller, and S. El Neil, "Outpatient Rehabilitative Treatment of Chronic Fatigue Syndrome (CFS/ME)," *Archives of Disease in Childhood* 89, no. 7 (2004): 615–19.

21. R. Viner, A. Gregorowski, C. Wine, M. Bladen, D. Fisher, M. Miller, and S. El Neil, "Outpatient Rehabilitative Treatment of Chronic Fatigue Syndrome (CFS/ME)," *Archives of Disease in Childhood* 89, no. 7 (2004): 615–19.

22. R. Viner R, A. Gregorowski, C. Wine, M. Bladen, D. Fisher, M. Miller, and S. El Neil, "Outpatient Rehabilitative Treatment of Chronic Fatigue Syndrome (CFS/ME)," *Archives of Disease in Childhood* 89, no. 7 (2004): 615–19.

23. Y. Gist and L. Hetzal, "We the People: Aging in the United States," U.S. Census Bureau, 2004, accessed July 4, 2014, www.census.gov/prod/2004pubs/censr-19.pdf.

24. B. Kozier, G. Erb, A. Berman, and S. Snyder, *Fundamentals of Nursing: Concepts, Process, and Practice*, 7th ed. (Singapore: Pearson Education South East Asia, 2004), 95.

25. B. Kozier, G. Erb, A. Berman, and S. Snyder, *Fundamentals of Nursing: Concepts, Process, and Practice*, 7th ed. (Singapore: Pearson Education South East Asia, 2004), 96.

26. H. Cho, P. Menezes, D. Bhugra, and S. Wessely, "The Awareness of Chronic Fatigue Syndrome: A Comparative Study in Brazil and the United Kingdom," *Journal of Psychosomatic Research* 64, no. 4 (2008): 351–55.

27. P. McCrone, L. Darbishire, L. Ridsdale, and P. Seed, "The Economic Cost of Chronic Fatigue and Chronic Fatigue Syndrome in UK Primary Care," *Psychological Medicine* 33, no. 2 (2003): 253–61.

28. B. Kozier, G. Erb, A. Berman, and S. Snyder, *Fundamentals of Nursing: Concepts, Process, and Practice*, 7th ed. (Singapore: Pearson Education South East Asia, 2004), 96.

29. B. Kozier, G. Erb, A. Berman, and S. Snyder, *Fundamentals of Nursing: Concepts, Process, and Practice*, 7th ed. (Singapore: Pearson Education South East Asia, 2004), 95.

30. J. Weissman, J. Ayanian, S. Chasan-Taber, M. Sherwood, C. Roth, and A. Epstein, "Hospital Readmissions and Quality of Care," *Medical Care* 37, no. 5 (1999): 490–501.

31. A. Deale and S. Wessely, "Patients' Perceptions of Medical Care in Chronic Fatigue Syndrome," *Social Science and Medicine* 52, no. 12 (2001): 1859–64.

32. A. Deale and S. Wessely, "Patients' Perceptions of Medical Care in Chronic Fatigue Syndrome," *Social Science and Medicine* 52, no. 12 (2001): 1859–64.

33. A. Deale and S. Wessely, "Patients' Perceptions of Medical Care in Chronic Fatigue Syndrome," *Social Science and Medicine* 52, no. 12 (2001): 1859–64.

34. A. Deale and S. Wessely, "Patients' Perceptions of Medical Care in Chronic Fatigue Syndrome," *Social Science and Medicine* 52, no. 12 (2001): 1859–64.

35. R. Webb, "Addressing the Global Health Work Force Crisis: Challenges for France, Germany, Italy, Spain and the UK," Action for Global Health 2011, accessed July 6, 2014, www.actionforglobalhealth.eu.

36. B. Kozier, G. Erb, A. Berman, and S. J. Snyder, *Fundamentals of Nursing: Concepts, Process, and Practice*, 7th ed. (Singapore: Pearson Education South East Asia, 2004), 94.

37. J. Penrod, P. Deb, C. Luhrs, C. Dellenbaugh, C. Zhu, T. Hochman, M. Maciejewski, E. Granieri, and R. Morrison, "Cost and Utilization Outcomes of Patients Receiving Hospital-based Palliative Care Consultation," *Journal of Palliative Medicine* 9, no. 4 (2006): 855–60.

38. B. Lucas, W. Trick, A. Evans, B. Mba, J. Smith, K. Das, P. Clarke, A. Varkey, S. Mathew, and R. Weinstein, "Effects of 2- vs. 4-week Attending Physician Inpatient Rotations on Unplanned Patient Revisits, Evaluations by Trainees, and Attending Physician Burnout: A Randomized Trial," *Journal of the American Medical Association* 308, no. 21 (2012): 2199–207.

39. C. Hawk, L. Jason, and S. Torres-Harding, "Differential Diagnosis of Chronic Fatigue Syndrome and Major Depressive Disorder," *International Journal of Behavioral Medicine* 13, no. 3 (2006): 244–51.

40. C. Blatch and T. Blatt, "Chronic Fatigue Syndrome: Role of Psychological Factors Overemphasised," *British Medical Journal* 308, no. 6939 (1994): 1297.

8. FATIGUE AND THE HUMAN BODY

1. H. Dong, I. Ugalde, N. Figueroa, and A. El-Saddik, "Towards Whole Body Fatigue Assessment of Human Movement: A Fatigue-tracking System Based on Combined sEMG and Accelerometer Signals," *Sensors* 14, no. 2 (2014): 2052–70.

2. C. Luca, "Myoelectrical Manifestations of Localized Muscular Fatigue in Humans," *CRC Critical Reviews in Biomedical Engineering* 11, no. 4 (1984): 251–79.

3. C. Luca, "Myoelectrical Manifestations of Localized Muscular Fatigue in Humans," *CRC Critical Reviews in Biomedical Engineering* 11, no. 4 (1984): 251–79.

4. National Collaborating Centre for Primary Care (UK), *Chronic Fatigue Syndrome/Myalgic Encephalomyelitis (or Encephalopathy): Diagnosis and Management of Chronic Fatigue Syndrome/Myalgic Encephalomyelitis (or Encephalopathy) in Adults and Children* (London: Royal College of General Practitioners, 2007).

5. H. Dong, I. Ugalde, N. Figueroa, and A. El-Saddik, "Towards Whole Body Fatigue Assessment of Human Movement: A Fatigue-tracking System Based on Combined sEMG and Accelerometer Signals," *Sensors* 14, no. 2 (2014): 2052–70.

6. H. Dong, I. Ugalde, N. Figueroa, and A. El-Saddik, "Towards Whole Body Fatigue Assessment of Human Movement: A Fatigue-tracking System Based on Combined sEMG and Accelerometer Signals," *Sensors* 14, no. 2 (2014): 2052–70.

7. R. Nardone, Y. Höller, F. Brigo, P. Höller, M. Christova, F. Tezzon, S. Golaszewski, and E. Trinka, "Fatigue-induced Motor Cortex Excitability Changes in Subjects with Spinal Cord Injury," *Brain Research Bulletin* 99 (2013): 9–12.

8. J. Davis, N. Anderson, and R. Welch, "Serotonin and Central Nervous System Fatigue: Nutritional Considerations," *American Journal for Clinical Nutrition* 72, Suppl. 2 (2000): 573S–578S.

9. A. Gualano, T. Bozza, P. Lopes De Campos, H. Roschel, A. Dos Santos Costa, M. Luiz Marquezi, F. Benatti, and A. Lancha Jr., "Branched-chain Amino Acids Supplementation Enhances Exercise Capacity and Lipid Oxidation during Endurance Exercise after Muscle Glycogen Depletion," *The Journal of Sports Medicine and Physical Fitness* 51, no. 1 (2011): 82–88.

10. A. Strachan and R. Maughan, "Platelet Serotonin Transporter Density and Related Parameters in Endurance-trained and Sedentary Male Subjects," *Acta Physiologica* 163, no. 2 (1998): 165–71.

11. E. Newsholme and E. Blomstrand, "Branched-chain Amino Acids and Central Fatigue," *Journal of Nutrition* 136, Suppl. 1 (2006): 274S–6S.

12. T. Friedman and C. Kimbal, "Endocrine Causes of Chronic Fatigue Syndrome (CFS)/Chronic Fatigue Immune: A Brief Guide for Primary Care Physicians," accessed May 23, 2014, www.goodhormonehealth.com/endo-causes.pdf.

13. K. Evans, D. Flanagan, and T. Wilkin, "Chronic Fatigue: Is It Endocrinology? *Clinical Medicine* 9, no. 1 (2009): 34–38.

14. K. Evans, D. Flanagan, and T. Wilkin, "Chronic Fatigue: Is It Endocrinology? *Clinical Medicine* 9, no. 1 (2009): 34–38.

15. J. Dempsey, M. Amann, L. Romer, and J. Miller, "Respiratory System Determinants of Peripheral Fatigue and Endurance Performance," *Medicine & Science in Sports & Exercise* 40, no. 3 (2008): 457–61.

16. J. Dempsey, M. Amann, L. Romer, and J. Miller, "Respiratory System Determinants of Peripheral Fatigue and Endurance Performance," *Medicine & Science in Sports & Exercise* 40, no. 3 (2008): 457–61.

17. J. Dempsey, M. Amann, L. Romer, and J. Miller, "Respiratory System Determinants of Peripheral Fatigue and Endurance Performance," *Medicine & Science in Sports & Exercise* 40, no. 3 (2008): 457–61.

18. J. Dempsey, M. Amann, L. Romer, and J. Miller, "Respiratory System Determinants of Peripheral Fatigue and Endurance Performance," *Medicine & Science in Sports & Exercise* 40, no. 3 (2008): 457–61.

19. B. Carruthers, A. Jain, K. De Meirleir, D. Peterson, N. Klimas, and A. Lerner, "Myalgic Encephalomyelitis/Chronic Fatigue Syndrome: Clinical Working Case Definition, Diagnostics, and Treatment Protocols," *Journal of Chronic Fatigue Syndrome* 11, no. 1 (2003): 7–36.

20. B. Carruthers, A. Jain, K. De Meirleir, D. Peterson, N. Klimas, and A. Lerner, "Myalgic Encephalomyelitis/Chronic Fatigue Syndrome: Clinical Working Case Definition, Diagnostics, and Treatment Protocols," *Journal of Chronic Fatigue Syndrome* 11, no. 1 (2003): 7–36.

21. B. Carruthers, A. Jain, K. De Meirleir, D. Peterson, N. Klimas, and A. Lerner, "Myalgic Encephalomyelitis/Chronic Fatigue Syndrome: Clinical Working Case Definition, Diagnostics, and Treatment Protocols," *Journal of Chronic Fatigue Syndrome* 11, no. 1 (2003): 7–36.

22. B. Carruthers, A. Jain, K. De Meirleir, D. Peterson, N. Klimas, and A. Lerner, "Myalgic Encephalomyelitis/Chronic Fatigue Syndrome: Clinical Working Case Definition, Diagnostics, and Treatment Protocols," *Journal of Chronic Fatigue Syndrome* 11, no. 1 (2003): 7–36.

23. S. Zakynthinos and C. Roussos, "Respiratory Muscle Fatigue," in *Physiologic Basis of Respiratory Disease*, ed. Q. Hamid, J. Shannon and J. Martin (Ontario, Canada: BC Decker Inc., 2005).

24. S. Zakynthinos and C. Roussos, "Respiratory Muscle Fatigue," in *Physiologic Basis of Respiratory Disease*, ed. Q. Hamid, J. Shannon, and J. Martin (Ontario, Canada: BC Decker Inc., 2005); J. Davis, N. Andeson, and R. Welch, "Serotonin and Central Nervous System Fatigue: Nutritional Considerations," *Americal Journal for Clincal Nutrition* 72, Suppl. 2 (2000): 573S–578S.

25. S. Zakynthinos and C. Roussos, "Respiratory Muscle Fatigue," in *Physiologic Basis of Respiratory Disease*, ed. Q. Hamid, J. Shannon, and J. Martin, (Ontario, Canada: BC Decker Inc., 2005); J. Davis, N. Andeson, and R. Welch, "Serotonin and Central Nervous System Fatigue: Nutritional Considerations," *Americal Journal for Clincal Nutrition* 72, Suppl. 2 (2000): 573S–578S.

26. M.-R. Huerta-Franco, M. Vargas-Luna, P. Tienda, I. Delgadillo-Holtfort, M. Balleza-Ordaz, and C. Flores-Hernandez, "Effects of Occupational Stress on the Gastrointestinal Tract," *World Journal of Gastrointestinal Pathophysiology* 4, no. 4 (2013): 108–18.

27. B. Carruthers, A. Jain, K. De Meirleir, D. Peterson, N. Klimas, and A. Lerner, "Myalgic Encephalomyelitis/Chronic Fatigue Syndrome: Clinical Working Case Definition, Diagnostics, and Treatment Protocols," *Journal of Chronic Fatigue Syndrome* 11, no. 1 (2003): 7–36.

28. K. Kahol, M. Smith, S. Mayes, M. Deka, V. Deka, J. Ferrara, and S. Panchanatan, "The Effects of Fatigue on Cognitive and Psychomotor Skills of Surgical Residents," 3rd International Conference on Foundation of Augmented Cognition (Heidelberg: Springer-Verlag Hesling, 2007), 304–13.

9. VIRAL, NEUROPSYCHIATRIC, AND NEUROENDOCRINE HYPOTHESES

1. P. Forterre, "The Origin of Viruses and their Possible Roles in Major Evolutionary Transitions," *Virus Research* 117, no. 1 (2006): 5–16.

2. E. Holmes, "What Does Virus Evolution Tell Us about Virus Origins?" *Journal of Virology* 85, no. 11 (2011): 5247–51.

3. E. Holmes, "What Does Virus Evolution Tell Us about Virus Origins?" *Journal of Virology* 85, no. 11 (2011): 5247–51.

4. C. Johnson, "One Theory to Explain Them All? The Vagus Nerve Infection Hypothesis for Chronic Fatigue Syndrome," Simmaron Research, accessed December 28, 2013, www.simmaronresearch.com/2013/12/one-theory-explain-vagus-nerve-infection-chronic-fatigue-syndrome/#sthash.hipkT6P6.dpuf.

5. M. Van Elzakker, "Chronic Fatigue Syndrome from Vagus Nerve Infection: A Psychoneuroimmunological Hypothesis," *Medical Hypotheses* 81, no. 3 (2013): 414–23.

6. M. Van Elzakker, "Chronic Fatigue Syndrome from Vagus Nerve Infection: A Psychoneuroimmunological Hypothesis," Medical Hypotheses 81, no. 3 (2013): 414–23.

7. C. Johnson, "One Theory to Explain Them All? The Vagus Nerve Infection Hypothesis for Chronic Fatigue Syndrome," Simmaron Research, accessed December 28, 2013, www.simmaronresearch.com/2013/12/one-theory-explain-vagus-nerve-infection-chronic-fatigue-syndrome/#sthash.hipkT6P6.dpuf.

8. C. Johnson, "One Theory to Explain Them All? The Vagus Nerve Infection Hypothesis for Chronic Fatigue Syndrome," Simmaron Research, accessed December 28, 2013, www.simmaronresearch.com/2013/12/one-theory-explain-vagus-nerve-infection-chronic-fatigue-syndrome/#sthash.hipkT6P6.dpuf.

9. C. Johnson, "One Theory to Explain Them All? The Vagus Nerve Infection Hypothesis for Chronic Fatigue Syndrome," Simmaron Research, accessed December 28, 2013, www.simmaronresearch.com/2013/12/one-theory-explain-vagus-nerve-infection-chronic-fatigue-syndrome/#sthash.hipkT6P6.dpuf.

10. C. Johnson, "One Theory to Explain Them All? The Vagus Nerve Infection Hypothesis for Chronic Fatigue Syndrome," Simmaron Research, accessed December 28, 2013, www.simmaronresearch.com/2013/12/one-theory-explain-vagus-nerve-infection-chronic-fatigue-syndrome/#sthash.hipkT6P6.dpuf.

11. G. Morris and M. Maes, "A Neuro-immune Model of Myalgic Encephalomyelitis/Chronic Fatigue Syndrome," *Metabolic Brain Disease* 28, no. 4 (2013): 523–40.

12. G. Morris and M. Maes, "Myalgic Encephalomyelitis/Chronic Fatigue Syndrome and Encephalomyelitis Disseminata/Multiple Sclerosis Show Remarkable Levels of Similarity in Phenomenology and Neuroimmune Characteristics," *BMC Medicine* 11 (2013): 205.

13. D. Schrijvers, F. Van Den Eede, Y. Maas, P. Cosyns, W. Hulstijn, and B. Sabbe, "Psychomotor Functioning in Chronic Fatigue Syndrome and Major Depressive Disorder: A Comparative Study," *Journal of Affective Disorders* 115, nos. 1–2 (2009): 46–53.

14. M. Maes, "Inflammatory and Oxidative and Nitrosative Stress Pathways Underpinning Chronic Fatigue, Somatization and Psychosomatic Symptoms," *Current Opinion in Psychiatry* 22, no. 1 (2009): 75–83.

15. E. Fuller-Thomson and J. Nimigon, "Factors Associated with Depression among Individuals with Chronic Fatigue Syndrome: Findings from a Nationally Representative Survey," *Family Practice* 25, no. 6 (2008): 414–22; M. Offenbaecher, K. Glatzeder, and M. Ackenheil, "Self-reported Depression, Familial History of Depression and Fibromyalgia (FM), and Psychological Distress in Patients with FM," *Zeitschrift für Rheumatologie* 57, Suppl. 2 (1998): 94–96; D. Buchwald, T. Pearlman, P. Kith, W. Katon, and K. Schmaling, "Screening for Psychiatric Disorders in Chronic Fatigue and Chronic Fatigue Syndrome," *Journal of Psychosomatic Research* 42, no. 1 (1997): 87–94; Y. Christley, T. Duffy, I. Everall, and C. Martin, "The Neuropsychiatric and Neuropsychological Features of Chronic Fatigue Syndrome: Revisiting the Enigma," *Current Psychiatry Reports* 15, no. 4 (2013): 353.

16. E. Fuller-Thomson and J. Nimigon, "Factors Associated with Depression among Individuals with Chronic Fatigue Syndrome: Findings from a Nationally Representative Survey," *Family Practice* 25, no. 6 (2008): 414–22; M. Offenbaecher, K. Glatzeder, and M. Ackenheil, "Self-reported Depression, Familial History of Depression and Fibromyalgia (FM), and Psychological Distress in Patients with FM," *Zeitschrift für Rheumatologie* 57, Suppl 2 (1998): 94–96; D. Buchwald, T. Pearlman, P. Kith, W. Katon, and K Schmaling, "Screening for Psychiatric Disorders in Chronic Fatigue and Chronic Fatigue Syndrome," *Journal of Psychosomatic Research* 42, no. 1 (1997): 87–94; Y. Christley, T. Duffy, I. Everall, and C. Martin, "The Neuropsychiatric and Neuropsychological Features of Chronic Fatigue Syndrome: Revisiting the Enigma," *Current Psychiatry Reports* 15, no. 4 (2013): 353.

17. L. Aaron, M. Burke, and D. Buchwald, "Overlapping Conditions among Patients with Chronic Fatigue Syndrome, Fibromyalgia, and Temporomandibular Disorder," *Archives of Internal Medicine* 160, no. 2 (2000): 221–27.

18. P. Sanders and J. Korf, "Neuroaetiology of Chronic Fatigue Syndrome: An Overview," *The World Journal of Biological Psychiatry* 9, no. 3 (2008): 165–71.

19. S. Johnson, J. DeLuca, and B. Natelson, "Depression in Fatiguing Illness: Comparing Patients with Chronic Fatigue Syndrome, Multiple Sclerosis and Depression," *Journal of Affective Disorders* 39, no. 1 (1996): 21–30.

20. S. Johnson, J. DeLuca, and B. Natelson, "Depression in Fatiguing Illness: Comparing Patients with Chronic Fatigue Syndrome, Multiple Sclerosis and Depression," *Journal of Affective Disorders* 39, no. 1 (1996): 21–30.

21. C. Hawk, L. Jason, and S. Torres-Harding, "Differential Diagnosis of Chronic Fatigue Syndrome and Major Depressive Disorder," *International Journal of Behavioral Medicine* 13, no. 3 (2006): 244–51.

22. E. Axe, P. Satz, N. Rasgon, and F. Fawzy, "Major Depressive Disorder in Chronic Fatigue Syndrome: A CDC Surveillance Study," *Journal of Chronic*

Fatigue Syndrome 12, no. 3 (2004): 7–23; L. Jason, J. Richman, F. Friedberg, L. Wagner, R. Taylor, and K. Jordan, "Politics, Science, and the Emergence of a New Disease, The Case of Chronic Fatigue Syndrome," *American Psychologist* 52, no. 9 (1997): 973–83.

23. A. Silver, M. Haeney, P. Vijayadurai, D. Wilks, M. Pattrick, and C. Main, "The Role of Fear of Physical Movement and Activity in Chronic Fatigue Syndrome," *Journal of Psychosomatic Research* 52, no. 6 (2002): 485–93.

24. E. Axe, P. Satz, N. Rasgon, and F. Fawzy, "Major Depressive Disorder in Chronic Fatigue Syndrome: A CDC Surveillance Study," *Journal of Chronic Fatigue Syndrome* 12, no. 3 (2004): 7–23.

25. B. Leonard and M. Maes, "Mechanistic Explanations How Cell-mediated Immune Activation, Inflammation and Oxidative and Nitrosative Stress Pathways and Their Sequels and Concomitants Play a Role in the Pathophysiology of Unipolar Depression," *Neuroscience and Biobehavioral Reviews* 36, no. 2 (2012): 764–85.

26. M. Maes, I. Mihaylova, and J. Leunis, "Increased Serum IgM Antibodies Directed against Phosphatidyl Inositol (Pi) in Chronic Fatigue Syndrome (CFS) and Major Depression: Evidence that an IgMmediated Immune Response against Pi Is One Factor Underpinning the Comorbidity between Both CFS and Depression," *Neuroendocrinology Letters* 28, no. 6 (2007): 861–67.

27. A. Roberts, A. Papadopoulos, S. Wessely, T. Chalder, and A. Cleare, "Salivary Cortisol Output before and after Cognitive Behavioural Therapy for Chronic Fatigue Syndrome," *Journal of Affective Disorders* 115, nos. 1–2 (2009): 280–86; A. Cleare, "The Neuroendocrinology of Chronic Fatigue Syndrome," *Endocrine Reviews* 24, no. 2 (2003): 236–52.

28. M. Maes and F. Twisk, "Chronic Fatigue Syndrome: Harvey and Wessely's (Bio)Psychosocial Model versus a Bio(Psychosocial) Model Based on Inflammatory and Oxidative and Nitrosative Stress Pathways," *Biomed Central Medicine* 8 (2010): 35.

29. K. Hinkelmann, S. Moritz, J. Botzenhardt, C. Muhtz, K. Wiedemann, M. Kellner, and C. Otte, "Changes in Cortisol Secretion during Antidepressive Treatment and Cognitive Improvement in Patients with Major Depression: A Longitudinal Study," *Psychoneuroendocrinology* 37, no. 5 (2011): 685–92.

30. K. Hinkelmann, S. Moritz, J. Botzenhardt, K. Riedesel, K. Wiedemann, and M. Kellner, "Cognitive Impairment in Major Depression: Association with Salivary Cortisol," *Biological Psychiatry* 66, no. 9 (2009): 879–85; R. Gomez, J. Posener, J. Keller, C. DeBattista, B. Solvason, and A. Schatzberg, "Effects of Major Depression Diagnosis and Cortisol Levels on Indices of Neurocognitive Function," *Psychoneuroendocrinology* 34, no. 7 (2009): 1012–18; A. Roberts, A. Papadopoulos, S. Wessely, T. Chalder, and A. Cleare, "Salivary Cortisol

Output before and after Cognitive Behavioral Therapy for Chronic Fatigue Syndrome," *Journal of Affective Disorders* 115, nos. 1–2 (2009): 280–86.

31. T. Turan, H. Izgi, S. Ozsoy, F. Tanriverdi, M. Basturk, and A. Asdemir, "The Effects of Galantamine Hydrobromide Treatment on Dehydroepiandrosterone Sulfate and Cortisol Levels in Patients with Chronic Fatigue Syndrome," *Psychiatry Investigation* 6, no. 3 (2009): 204–10.

32. L. Parker, E. Levin, and E. Lifrak, "Evidence for Adrenocortical Adaptation to Severe Illness," *The Journal of Clinical Endocrinology and Metabolism* 60, no. 5 (1985): 947–52.

33. L. Scott, F. Svec, and T. Dinan, "A Preliminary Study of Dehydroepiandrosterone Response to Low-dose ACTH in Chronic Fatigue Syndrome and in Healthy Subjects," *Psychiatric Research* 97, no. 1 (2000): 21–28.

34. P. Himmel and T. Seligman, "A Pilot Study Employing Dehydroepiandrosterone (DHEA) in the Treatment of Chronic Fatigue Syndrome," *Journal of Clinical Rheumatology* 5, no. 2 (1999): 56–59.

35. P. Manu, G. Affleck, H. Tennen, P. Morse, and J. Escobar, "Hypochondriasis Influences Quality-of-life Outcomes in Patients with Chronic Fatigue," *Psychotherapy and Psychosomatics* 65, no. 2 (1996): 76–81.

36. C. Pepper, L. Krupp, F. Friedberg, C. Doscher, and P. Coyle, "A Comparison of Neuropsychiatric Characteristics in Chronic Fatigue Syndrome, Multiple Sclerosis, and Major Depression," *The Journal of Neuropsychiatry and Clinical Neurosciences* 5, no. 2 (1993): 200–205.

37. B. Fischler, P. Dendale, V. Michiels, R. Cluydts, L. Kaufman, and K. De Meirleir, "Physical Fatigability and Exercise Capacity in Chronic Fatigue Syndrome: Association with Disability, Somatization and Psychopathology," *Journal of Psychosomatic Research* 42, no. 4 (1997): 369–78.

38. B. Fischler, P. Dendale, V. Michiels, R. Cluydts, L. Kaufman, and K. De Meirleir, "Physical Fatigability and Exercise Capacity in Chronic Fatigue Syndrome: Association with Disability, Somatization and Psychopathology," *Journal of Psychosomatic Research* 42, no. 4 (1997): 369–78.

39. Z. Lipowski, "Somatization: The Concept and Its Clinical Application," *American Journal of Psychiatry* 145 (1988): 1358–68.

40. L. Kirmayer, J. Robbins, and J. Paris, "Somatoform Disorders: Personality and the Social Matrix of Somatic Distress," *Journal of Abnormal Psychology* 103, no. 1 (1994): 125–36.

41. S. Abbey, "Somatization, Illness Attribution and the Sociocultural Psychiatry of Chronic Fatigue Syndrome," *Ciba Foundation Symposium* 173 (1993): 238–52.

42. C. Pepper, B. Krupp, F. Friedberg, C. Doscher, and P. Coyle, "A Comparison of Neuropsychiatric Characteristics in Chronic Fatigue Syndrome, Multiple Sclerosis, and Major Depression," *The Journal of Neuropsychiatry*

and Clinical Neurosciences 5, no. 2 (1993): 200–205; S. Johnson, J. DeLuca, and B. Natelson, "Assessing Somatization Disorder in the Chronic Fatigue Syndrome," *Psychosomatic Medicine* 58, no. 1 (1996): 50–57; P. Manu, T. Lane, D. Matthews, and J. Escobar, "Screening for Somatization Disorder in Patients with Chronic Fatigue," *General Hospital Psychiatry* 11 (1989): 294–97; S. Johnson, J. DeLuca, and B. Natelson, "Assessing Somatization Disorder in the Chronic Fatigue Syndrome," *Psychosomatic Medicine* 58, no. 1 (1996): 50–57.

43. J. Johnson, J. DeLuca, and B. Natelson, "Assessing Somatization Disorder in the Chronic Fatigue Syndrome," *Psychosomatic Medicine* 58, no. 1 (1996): 50–57.

44. M. Demitrack, "Neuroendocrine Research Strategies in Chronic Fatigue Syndrome," in *Chronic Fatigue and Related Immune Deficiency Syndromes*, ed. P. Goodnick and N. Klimas (Washington: American Psychiatric Press, 1993), 45–66.

45. W. Katon and E. Walker, "The Relationship of Chronic Fatigue to Psychiatric Illness in Community, Primary Care and Tertiary Care Samples," *Ciba Foundation Symposium* 173, no. (1993): 193–204.

46. W. Katon and J. Russo, "Chronic Fatigue Syndrome Criteria: A Critique of the Requirement for Multiple Physical Complaints," *Archives of Internal Medicine* 152, no. 8 (1992): 1604–9.

47. S. Johnson, J. DeLuca, and B. Natelson, "Personality Dimensions in the Chronic Fatigue Syndrome: A Comparison with Multiple Sclerosis and Depression," *Journal of Psychiatric Research* 30, no. 1 (1996): 9–20.

48. S. Johnson, J. DeLuca, and B. Natelson, "Personality Dimensions in the Chronic Fatigue Syndrome: A Comparison with Multiple Sclerosis and Depression," *Journal of Psychiatric Research* 30, no. 1 (1996): 9–20.

49. S. Johnson, J. DeLuca, and B. Natelson, "Personality Dimensions in the Chronic Fatigue Syndrome: A Comparison with Multiple Sclerosis and Depression," *Journal of Psychiatric Research* 30, no. 1 (1996): 9–20.

50. J. Deluca, C. Christodoulou, B. Diamond, E. Rosenstein, N. Kramer, and B. Natelson, "Working Memory Deficits in Chronic Fatigue Syndrome: Differentiating between Speed and Accuracy of Information Processing," *Journal of the International Neuropsychological Society* 10, no. 1 (2004): 101–9.

51. M. Majer, L. Welberg, L. Capuron, A. Miller, G. Pagnoni, and W. Reeves, "Neuropsychological Performance in Persons with Chronic Fatigue Syndrome: Results from a Population-based Study," *Psychosomatic Medicine* 70, no. 7 (2008): 829–36; A. Wearden and L. Appleby, "Cognitive Performance and Complaints of Cognitive Impairment in Chronic Fatigue Syndrome (CFS)," *Psychological Medicine* 27, no. 1 (1997): 81–90.

52. M. Majer, L. Welberg, L. Capuron, A. Miller, G. Pagnoni, and W. Reeves, "Neuropsychological Performance in Persons with Chronic Fatigue Syndrome: Results from a Population-based Study," *Psychosomatic Medicine* 70, no. 7 (2008): 829–36.

53. S. Lutgendorf, M. Antoni, G. Ironson, M. Fletcher, F. Penedo, A. Baum, N. Schniederman, and N. Klimas, "Physical Symptoms of Chronic Fatigue Syndrome Are Exacerbated by the Stress of Hurricane Andrew," *Psychosomatic Medicine* 57, no. 4 (1995): 310–23.

54. V. Michiels and R. Cluydts, "Neuropsychological Functioning in Chronic Fatigue Syndrome: A Review," *Acta Psychiatrica Scandinavica* 103, no. 2 (2001): 84–93.

55. V. Michiels and R. Cluydts, "Neuropsychological Functioning in Chronic Fatigue Syndrome: A Review," *Acta Psychiatrica Scandinavica* 103, no. 2 (2001): 84–93; L. Tiersky, S. Johnson, G. Lange, B. Natelson, and J. DeLuca, "Neuropsychology of Chronic Fatigue Syndrome: A Critical Review," *Journal of Clinical and Experimental Neuropsychology* 19, no. 4 (1997): 560–86.

56. R. Mahurin, K. Claypoole, J. Goldberg, L. Arguelles, S. Ashton, and D. Buchwald, "Cognitive Processing in Monozygotic Twins Discordant for Chronic Fatigue Syndrome," Neuropsychology 18, no. 2 (2004): 232–39; J. Deluca, C. Christodoulou, B. Diamond, E. Rosenstein, N. Kramer, and B. Natelson, "Working Memory Deficits in Chronic Fatigue Syndrome: Differentiating between Speed and Accuracy of Information Processing," *Journal of the International Neuropsychological Society* 10, no. 1 (2004): 101–9; M. Majer, L. Welberg, L. Capuron, A. Miller, G. Pagnoni, and W. Reeves, "Neuropsychological Performance in Persons with Chronic Fatigue Syndrome: Results from a Population-based Study," *Psychosomatic Medicine* 70, no. 7 (2008): 829–36; L. Capuron, L. Welberg, C. Heim, D. Wagner, L. Solomon, D. Papanicolaou, R. Craddock, A. Miller, and W. Reeves, "Cognitive Dysfunction Relates to Subjective Report of Mental Fatigue in Patients with Chronic Fatigue Syndrome," *Neuropsychopharmacology* 31, no. 8 (2006): 1777–84.

57. S. Crowe and A. Casey, "A Neuropsychological Study of the Chronic Fatigue Syndrome: Support for a Deficit in Memory Function Independent of Depression," *Australian Psychological Society* 34, no. 1 (1999): 70–75; N. Fiedler, H. Kipen, J. DeLuca, K. Kelly-McNeil, and B. Natelson, "Controlled Comparison of Multiple Chemical Sensitivities and Chronic Fatigue Syndrome," *Psychosomatic Medicine* 58, no. 1 (1996): 38–49.

58. V. Michiels and R. Cluydts, "Neuropsychological Functioning in Chronic Fatigue Syndrome: A Review," *Acta Psychiatrica Scandinavica* 103, no. 2 (2001): 84–93; L. Tiersky, S. Johnson, G. Lange, B. Natelson, and J. DeLuca, "Neuropsychology of Chronic Fatigue Syndrome: A Critical Review," *Journal of Clinical and Experimental Neuropsychology* 19, no. 4 (1997): 560–86.

59. S. Cockshell and J. Mathias, "Cognitive Functioning in Chronic Fatigue Syndrome: A Meta-Analysis," *Psychological Medicine* 40, no. 8 (2010): 1253–67; J. Deluca, C. Christodoulou, B. Diamond, E. Rosenstein, N. Kramer, and B. Natelson, "Working Memory Deficits in Chronic Fatigue Syndrome: Differentiating between Speed and Accuracy of Information Processing," *Journal of the International Neuropsychological Society* 10, no. 1 (2004): 101–9; M. Majer, L. Welberg, L. Capuron, A. Miller, G. Pagnoni, and W. Reeves, "Neuropsychological Performance in Persons with Chronic Fatigue Syndrome: Results from a Population-based Study," *Psychosomatic Medicine* 70, no. 7 (2008): 829–36; L. Tiersky, R. Matheis, J. Deluca, G. Lange, B. Natelson, "Functional Status, Neuropsychological Functioning, and Mood in Chronic Fatigue Syndrome (CFS): Relationship to Psychiatric Disorder," *The Journal of Nervous and Mental Disease* 191, no. 5 (2003): 324–31.

60. J. Deluca, C. Christodoulou, B. Diamond, E. Rosenstein, N. Kramer, and B. Natelson, "Working Memory Deficits in Chronic Fatigue Syndrome: Differentiating between Speed and Accuracy of Information Processing," *Journal of the International Neuropsychological Society* 10, no. 1 (2004): 101–9.

61. J. Deluca, C. Christodoulou, B. Diamond, E. Rosenstein, N. Kramer, and B. Natelson, "Working Memory Deficits in Chronic Fatigue Syndrome: Differentiating between Speed and Accuracy of Information Processing," *Journal of the International Neuropsychological Society* 10, no. 1 (2004): 101–9.

62. F. Duffy, G. McAnulty, M. McCreary, G. Cuchural, and A. Komaroff, "EEG Spectral Coherence Data Distinguish Chronic Fatigue Syndrome Patients from Healthy Controls and Depressed Patients—A Case Control Study," BioMed Central Neurology 11 (2011): 82.

63. X. Caseras, D. Mataix-Cols, V. Giampietro, K. Rimes, M. Brammer, F. Zelaya, T. Chalder, and E. Godfrey, "Probing the Working Memory System in Chronic Fatigue Syndrome: A Functional Magnetic Resonance Imaging Study Using the N-back Task," *Psychosomatic Medicine* 68, no. 6 (2006): 947–55.

64. X. Caseras, D. Mataix-Cols, V. Giampietro, K. Rimes, M. Brammer, F. Zelaya, T. Chalder, and E. Godfrey, "Probing the Working Memory System in Chronic Fatigue Syndrome: A Functional Magnetic Resonance Imaging Study Using the N-back Task," *Psychosomatic Medicine* 68, no. 6 (2006): 947–55; K. Claypoole, C. Noonan, R. Mahurin, J. Goldberg, T. Erickson, and D. Buchwald, "A Twin Study of Cognitive Function in Chronic Fatigue Syndrome: The Effects of Sudden Illness Onset," *Neuropsychology* 21, no. 4 (2007): 507–13; R. Mahurin, K. Claypoole, J. Goldberg, L. Arguelles, S. Ashton, and D. Buchwald, "Cognitive Processing in Monozygotic Twins Discordant for Chronic Fatigue Syndrome," *Neuropsychology* 18, no. 2 (2004): 232–39; J. Deluca, C. Christodoulou, B. Diamond, E. Rosenstein, N. Kramer, and B. Natelson, "Working Memory Deficits in Chronic Fatigue Syndrome: Differentiating be-

tween Speed and Accuracy of Information Processing," *Journal of the International Neuropsychological Society* 10, no. 1 (2004): 101–9; N. Chiaravalloti, C. Christodoulou, H. Demaree, and J. DeLuca, "Differentiating Simple versus Complex Processing Speed: Influence on New Learning and Memory Performance," *Journal of Clinical and Experimental Neuropsychology* 25, no. 4 (2003): 489–501.

65. M. Kaplan, "Neuroendocrine Abnormalities in CFS Deserve More Comprehensive Study," Chronic Neuroimmune Diseases, last updated January 1, 2014, accessed June 3, 2014, www.anapsid.org/cnd/diagnosis/neuro.html.

66. A. Kavelaars, W. Kuis, L. Knook, G. Sinnema, and C. Heijnen, "Disturbed Neuroendocrine-immune Interactions in Chronic Fatigue Syndrome," *The Journal of Clinical Endocrinology and Metabolism* 85, no. 2 (2000): 692–96.

67. D. Buchwald, M. Wener, T. Pearlman, and P. Kith, "Markers of Inflammation and Immune Activation in Chronic Fatigue and Chronic Fatigue Syndrome," *The Journal of Rheumatology* 24, no. 2 (1997): 372–76.

68. A. Kavelaars, W. Kuis, L. Knook, G. Sinnema, and C. Heijnen, "Disturbed Neuroendocrine-immune Interactions in Chronic Fatigue Syndrome," *The Journal of Clinical Endocrinology & Metabolism* 85, no. 2 (2000): 692–96.

69. J. Gaab, N. Rohleder, V. Heitz, V. Engert, T. Schad, T. Schürmeyer, and U. Ehlert, "Stress-induced Changes in LPS-induced Pro-inflammatory Cytokine Production in Chronic Fatigue Syndrome," *Psychoneuroendocrinology* 30, no. 2 (2005): 188–98.

70. M. Kaplan, "Neuroendocrine Abnormalities in CFS Deserve More Comprehensive Study," Chronic Neuroimmune Diseases, last updated January 1, 2014, accessed June 3, 2014, www.anapsid.org/cnd/diagnosis/neuro.html.

71. L. Scott, S. Medbak, and T. Dinan, "Blunted Adrenocorticotropin and Cortisol Responses to Corticotropin-releasing Hormone Stimulation in Chronic Fatigue Syndrome," *Acta Psychiatrica Scandinavica* 97, no. 6 (1998): 450–57.

72. M. Kaplan, "Neuroendocrine Abnormalities in CFS Deserve More Comprehensive Study," Chronic Neuroimmune Diseases, last updated January 1, 2014, accessed June 3, 2014, www.anapsid.org/cnd/diagnosis/neuro.html.

73. M. Kaplan, "Neuroendocrine Abnormalities in CFS Deserve More Comprehensive Study," Chronic Neuroimmune Diseases, last updated January 1, 2014, accessed June 3, 2014, www.anapsid.org/cnd/diagnosis/neuro.html.

74. T. Gerrity, D. Papanicolaou, J. Amsterdam, S. Bingham, A. Grossman, T. Hedrick, R. Herberman, G. Krueger, S. Levine, N. Mohagheghpour, R. Moore, J. Oleske, and C. Snell, "Immunologic Aspects of Chronic Fatigue Syndrome. Report on a Research Symposium Convened by The CFIDS Association of America and Co-sponsored by the U.S. Centers for Disease Control

and Prevention and the National Institutes of Health," *Neuroimmunomodulation* 11, no. 6 (2004): 351–57.

10. NATURAL APPROACHES TO CHRONIC FATIGUE SYNDROME

1. E. Weatherley-Jones, J. Nicholl, K. Thomas, G. Parry, M. McKendrick, S. Green, P. Stanley, and S. Lynch, "A Randomised, Controlled, Triple-blind Trial of the Efficacy of Homeopathic Treatment for Chronic Fatigue Syndrome," *Journal of Psychosomatic Research* 56, no. 2 (2004): 189–97.

2. E. Weatherley-Jones, J. Nicholl, K. Thomas, G. Parry, M. McKendrick, S. Green, P. Stanley, and S. Lynch, "A Randomised, Controlled, Triple-blind Trial of the Efficacy of Homeopathic Treatment for Chronic Fatigue Syndrome," *Journal of Psychosomatic Research* 56, no. 2 (2004): 189–97.

3. N. Porter, L. Jason, A. Boulton, N. Bothne, and B. Coleman, "Alternative Medical Interventions Used in the Treatment and Management of Myalgic Encephalomyelitis/Chronic Fatigue Syndrome and Fibromyalgia," *Journal of Alternative and Complementary Medicine* 16, no. 3 (2010): 235–49.

4. A. Hartz, S. Bentler, R. Noyes, J. Hoehns, C. Logemann, S. Sinift, Y. Butani, W. Wang, K. Brake, M. Ernst, and H. Kautzman, "Randomized Controlled Trial of Siberian Ginseng for Chronic Fatigue," *Psychological Medicine* 34, no. 1 (2004): 51–61.

5. J. Sarris, S. Moylan, D. Camfield, M. Pase, D. Mischoulon, M. Berk, F. Jacka, and I. Schweitzer, "Complementary Medicine, Exercise, Meditation, Diet, and Lifestyle Modification for Anxiety Disorders: A Review of Current Evidence," *Evidence Based Complementary and Alternative Medicine* 2012 (2012): 809653.

6. S. McDowell, H. Ferner, and R. Ferner, "The Pathophysiology of Medication Errors: How and Where They Arise," *British Journal of Clinical Pharmacology* 67, no. 6 (2009): 605–13.

7. M. Hooper, "Myalgic Encephalomyelitis: A Review with Emphasis on Key Findings in Biomedical Research," *Journal of Clinical Pathology* 60, no. 5 (2007): 466–71.

8. L. Borish, K. Schmaling, J. DiClementi, J. Streib, J. Negri, and J. Jones, "Chronic Fatigue Syndrome: Identification of Distinct Subgroups on the Basis of Allergy and Psychologic Variables," *Journal of Allergy and Clinical Immunology* 102, no. 2 (1998): 222–30.

9. J. Vercoulen, C. Swanink, J. Fennis, J. Galama, J. van der Meer, and G. Bleijenberg, "Prognosis in Chronic Fatigue Syndrome: A Prospective Study on the Natural Course," *Journal of Neurology, Neurosurgery & Psychiatry* 60, no. 5 (1996): 489–94.

10. J. Vercoulen, C. Swanink, J. Fennis, J. Galama, J. van der Meer, and G. Bleijenberg, "Prognosis in Chronic Fatigue Syndrome: A Prospective Study on the Natural Course," *Journal of Neurology, Neurosurgery & Psychiatry* 60, no. 5 (1996): 489–94.

11. A. Singh, P. Naidu, S. Gupta, and S. Kulkarni, "Effect of Natural and Synthetic Antioxidants in a Mouse Model of Chronic Fatigue Syndrome," *Journal of Medicinal Food* 5, no. 4 (2002): 211–20.

12. J. Bamidele, W. Adebimpe, and E. Oladele, "Knowledge, Attitude and Use of Alternative Medical Therapy amongst Urban Residents of Osun State, Southwestern Nigeria," *African Journal of Traditional, Complementary, and Alternative Medicines* 6, no. 3 (2009): 281–88.

13. B. Voerman, A. Visser, M. Fischer, B. Garssen, G. van Andel, and J. Bensing, "Determinants of Participation in Social Support Groups for Prostate Cancer Patients," *Psychooncology* 16, no. 12 (2007): 1092–99.

14. D. Locker, "Social Determinants of Health and Disease," in *Sociology As Applied to Medicine* (New York: Elselvier, 2008).

15. B. Van Houdenhove, E. Neerinckx, P. Onghena, A. Vingerhoets, R. Lysens, and H. Vertommen, "Daily Hassles Reported by Chronic Fatigue Syndrome and Fibromyalgia Patients in Tertiary Care: A Controlled Quantitative and Qualitative Study," *Psychotherapy and Psychosomatics* 71, no. 4 (2002): 207–13.

16. B. Van Houdenhove, E. Neerinckx, P. Onghena, A. Vingerhoets, R. Lysens, and H. Vertommen, "Daily Hassles Reported by Chronic Fatigue Syndrome and Fibromyalgia Patients in Tertiary Care: A Controlled Quantitative and Qualitative Study," *Psychotherapy and Psychosomatics* 71, no. 4 (2002): 207–13.

17. D. Chambers, A.-M. Bagnall, S. Hempel, and C. Forbes, "Interventions for the Treatment, Management and Rehabilitation of Patients with Chronic Fatigue Syndrome/Myalgic Encephalomyelitis: An Updated Systematic Review," *Journal of the Royal Society of Medicine* 99, no. 10 (2006): 506–20.

18. D. Chambers, A.-M. Bagnall, S. Hempel, and C. Forbes, "Interventions for the Treatment, Management and Rehabilitation of Patients with Chronic Fatigue Syndrome/Myalgic Encephalomyelitis: An Updated Systematic Review," *Journal of the Royal Society of Medicine* 99, no. 10 (2006): 506–20.

19. K. Schmaling, W. Smith, and D. Buchwald, "Significant Other Responses Are Associated with Fatigue and Functional Status among Patients with Chronic Fatigue Syndrome," *Psychosomatic Medicine* 62, no. 3 (2000): 444–50.

20. F. Friedberg, D. Leung, and J. Quick, "Do Support Groups Help People with Chronic Fatigue Syndrome and Fibromyalgia? A Comparison of Ac-

tive and Inactive Members," *Journal of Rheumatology* 32, no. 12 (2005): 2416–20.

21. F. Friedberg, D. Leung, and J. Quick, "Do Support Groups Help People with Chronic Fatigue Syndrome and Fibromyalgia? A Comparison of Active and Inactive Members," *Journal of Rheumatology* 32, no. 12 (2005): 2416–20.

22. J. Colby, "Special Problems of Children with Myalgic Encephalomyelitis/Chronic Fatigue Syndrome and the Enteroviral Link," *Journal of Clinical Pathology* 60, no. 2 (2007): 125–28.

23. J. Colby, "Special Problems of Children with Myalgic Encephalomyelitis/Chronic Fatigue Syndrome and the Enteroviral Link," *Journal of Clinical Pathology* 60, no. 2 (2007): 125–28.

24. J. Nijs, N. Roussel, J. Van-Oosterwijck, M. De-Kooning, K. Ickmans, F. Struyf, M. Meeus, and M. Lundberg, "Fear of Movement and Avoidance Behaviour toward Physical Activity in Chronic-Fatigue Syndrome and Fibromyalgia: State of the Art and Implications for Clinical Practice," *Clinical Rheumatology* 32, no. 8 (2013).

25. K. Schmaling, W. Smith, and D. Buchwald, "Significant Other Responses Are Associated with Fatigue and Functional Status among Patients with Chronic Fatigue Syndrome," *Psychosomatic Medicine* 62, no. 3 (2000): 444–50.

26. D. Chambers, A.-M. Bagnall, S. Hempel, and C. Forbes, "Interventions for the Treatment, Management and Rehabilitation of Patients with Chronic Fatigue Syndrome/Myalgic Encephalomyelitis: An Updated Systematic Review," *Journal of the Royal Society of Medicine* 99, no. 10 (2006): 506–20.

27. D. Chambers, A.-M. Bagnall, S. Hempel, and C. Forbes, "Interventions for the Treatment, Management and Rehabilitation of Patients with Chronic Fatigue Syndrome/Myalgic Encephalomyelitis: An Updated Systematic Review," *Journal of the Royal Society of Medicine* 99, no. 10 (2006): 506–20.

28. D. Chambers, A.-M. Bagnall, S. Hempel, and C. Forbes, "Interventions for the Treatment, Management and Rehabilitation of Patients with Chronic Fatigue Syndrome/Myalgic Encephalomyelitis: An Updated Systematic Review," *Journal of the Royal Society of Medicine* 99, no. 10 (2006).

29. A. Deale, T. Chalder, I. Marks, and S. Wessely, "Cognitive Behavior Therapy for Chronic Fatigue Syndrome: A Randomized Controlled Trial," *American Journal of Psychiatry* 154, no. 3 (1997).

30. D. Chambers, A.-M. Bagnall, S. Hempel, and C. Forbes, "Interventions for the Treatment, Management and Rehabilitation of Patients with Chronic Fatigue Syndrome/Myalgic Encephalomyelitis: An Updated Systematic Review," *Journal of the Royal Society of Medicine* 99, no. 10 (2006): 506–20.

31. D. Locker, "Social Determinants of Health and Disease," in *Sociology As Applied to Medicine* (New York: Elselvier, 2008).

32. D. Locker, "Social Determinants of Health and Disease," in *Sociology As Applied to Medicine* (New York: Elselvier, 2008).

33. D. Racciatti, J. Vecchiet, A. Ceccomancini, F. Ricci, and E. Pizzigallo, "Chronic Fatigue Syndrome Following a Toxic Exposure," *Science of the Total Environment* 270, no. 103 (2001): 27–31.

34. D. Racciatti, J. Vecchiet, A. Ceccomancini, F. Ricci, and E. Pizzigallo, "Chronic Fatigue Syndrome Following a Toxic Exposure," *Science of the Total Environment* 270, no. 103 (2001): 27–31.

35. D. Racciatti, J. Vecchiet, A. Ceccomancini, F. Ricci, and E. Pizzigallo, "Chronic Fatigue Syndrome Following a Toxic Exposure," *Science of the Total Environment* 270, no. 103 (2001): 27–31.

36. D. Racciatti, J. Vecchiet, A. Ceccomancini, F. Ricci, and E. Pizzigallo, "Chronic Fatigue Syndrome Following a Toxic Exposure," *Science of the Total Environment* 270, no. 103 (2001): 27–31.

37. E. Weatherley-Jones, J. Nicholl, K. Thomas, G. Parry, M. McKendrick, S. Green, P. Stanley, and S. Lynch, "A Randomised, Controlled, Triple-Blind Trial of the Efficacy of Homeopathic Treatment for Chronic Fatigue Syndrome," *Journal of Psychosomatic Research* 56, no. 2 (2004): 189–97; R. Awdry, "Homeopathy May Help Me," *The Journal of Alternative and Complementary Medicine* 14, no. 3 (1996): 12–16.

38. T. Alraek, M. Lee, T.-Y. Choi, H. Cao, and J. Liu, "Complementary and Alternative Medicine for Patients with Chronic Fatigue Syndrome: A Systematic Review," *BMC Complementary and Alternative Medicine* 11, no. 1 (2011): 87.

39. D. Grimes, "Proposed Mechanisms for Homeopathy Are Physically Impossible," *Focus on Alternative and Complementary Therapies* 17, no. 3 (2012): 149–55.

40. S. Kayne, *Homeopathic Pharmacy: Theory and Practice* (New York: Elsevier Health Sciences, 2006).

41. S. Kayne, *Homeopathic Pharmacy: Theory and Practice* (New York: Elsevier Health Sciences, 2006).

42. R. Hobday, S. Thomas, A. O'Donovan, M. Murphy, and A. Pinching, "Dietary Intervention in Chronic Fatigue Syndrome," *Journal of Human Nutrition and Dietetics* 21, no. 2 (2008): 141–49.

43. F. Kobayashi, H. Ogata, N. Omi, S. Nagasaka, S. Yamaguchi, M. Hibi, and K. Tokuyama, "Effect of Breakfast Skipping on Diurnal Variation of Energy Metabolism and Blood Glucose," *Obesity Research & Clinical Practice* 8, no. 3 (2014): e201–98.

44. K. Tandel, "Sugar Substitutes: Health Controversy over Perceived Benefits," *Journal of Pharmacology and Pharmacotherapeutics* 2, no. 4 (2011): 236–43.

45. K. Dykman, C. Tone, C. Ford, and R. Dykman, "The Effects of Nutritional Supplements on the Symptoms of Fibromyalgia and Chronic Fatigue Syndrome," *Integrative Physiological and Behavioral Science* 33, no. 1 (1998): 61–71.

46. G. Kumar and F. Khanum, "Neuroprotective Potential of Phytochemicals," *Pharmacognosy Reviews* 6, no. 12 (2012): 81–90.

47. A. Plioplys and S. Plioplys, "Amantadine and L-carnitine Treatment of Chronic Fatigue Syndrome," *Neuropsychobiology* 35, no. 1 (1997): 16–23.

48. M. Werbach, "Nutritional Strategies for Treating Chronic Fatigue Syndrome," *Alternative Medicine Review* 5, no. 2 (2000): 93–108.

49. A. Plioplys and S. Plioplys, "Amantadine and L-Carnitine Treatment of Chronic Fatigue Syndrome," *Neuropsychobiology* 35, no. 1 (1997): 16–23.

50. D. Chambers, A.-M. Bagnall, S. Hempel, and C. Forbes, "Interventions for the Treatment, Management and Rehabilitation of Patients with Chronic Fatigue Syndrome/Myalgic Encephalomyelitis: An Updated Systematic Review," *Journal of the Royal Society of Medicine* 99, no. 10 (2006): 506–20.

51. M. Werbach, "Nutritional Strategies for Treating Chronic Fatigue Syndrome," *Alternative Medicine Review* 5, no. 2 (2000): 93–108.

52. R. Hobday, S. Thomas, A. O'Donovan, M. Murphy, and A. Pinching, "Dietary Intervention in Chronic Fatigue Syndrome," *Journal of Human Nutrition and Dietetics* 21, no. 2 (2008): 141–49.

53. M. Werbach, "Nutritional Strategies for Treating Chronic Fatigue Syndrome," *Alternative Medicine Review* 5, no. 2 (2000): 93–108.

54. M. Werbach, "Nutritional Strategies for Treating Chronic Fatigue Syndrome," *Alternative Medicine Review* 5, no. 2 (2000): 93–108.

55. M. Werbach, "Nutritional Strategies for Treating Chronic Fatigue Syndrome," *Alternative Medicine Review* 5, no. 2 (2000): 93–108.

56. D. Maric, S. Brkic, A. Mikic, S. Tomic, T. Cebovic, and V. Turkulov, "Multivitamin Mineral Supplementation in Patients with Chronic Fatigue Syndrome," *Medical Science Monitor* 20 (2014): 47–53.

57. C. Lapp, "Q: Given the Complexities and Diversity of Symptoms of Cfids, How Do You Approach the Treatment of Cfids Patients?" (paper presented at the CFIDS Chronicle Physicians' Forum, 1991); F. Ellis and S. Nasser, "A Pilot Study of Vitamin B12 in the Treatment of Tiredness," *British Journal of Nutrition* 30, no. 2 (1973): 277–83; H. Newbold, "Vitamin B-12: Placebo or Neglected Therapeutic Tool?" *Medical Hypotheses* 28, no. 3 (1989): 155–64.

58. J. Kaslow, L. Rucker, and R. Onishi, "Liver Extract–Folic Acid–Cyanocobalamin vs. Placebo for Chronic Fatigue Syndrome," *Archives of Internal Medicine* 149, no. 11 (1989): 2501–3.

59. M. Werbach, "Nutritional Strategies for Treating Chronic Fatigue Syndrome," *Alternative Medicine Review* 5, no. 2 (2000): 93–108.

60. M. Werbach, "Nutritional Strategies for Treating Chronic Fatigue Syndrome," *Alternative Medicine Review* 5, no. 2 (2000): 93–108.

61. M. Werbach, "Nutritional Strategies for Treating Chronic Fatigue Syndrome," *Alternative Medicine Review* 5, no. 2 (2000): 93–108.

62. R. Cater II, "Chronic Intestinal Candidiasis As a Possible Etiological Factor in the Chronic Fatigue Syndrome," *Medical Hypotheses* 44, no. 6 (1995): 507–15.

63. R. Hobday, S. Thomas, A. O'Donovan, M. Murphy, and A. Pinching, "Dietary Intervention in Chronic Fatigue Syndrome," *Journal of Human Nutrition and Dietetics* 21, no. 2 (2008): 141–49.

64. L. Wilson, "Chronic Fatigue Syndrome," accessed May 13, 2014, www.drlwilson.com/Articles/chronic%20fatigue.htm.

65. M. Shilstone, *Maximum Energy for Life: A 21-Day Strategic Plan to Feel Great, Reverse the Aging Process, and Optimize Your Health* (Hoboken, NJ: John Wiley & Sons, 2003).

66. M. Timlin and M. Pereira, "Breakfast Frequency and Quality in the Etiology of Adult Obesity and Chronic Diseases," *Nutrition Reviews* 65, no. 6 (2007): 268–81.

67. M. Timlin and M. Pereira, "Breakfast Frequency and Quality in the Etiology of Adult Obesity and Chronic Diseases," *Nutrition Reviews* 65, no. 6 (2007): 268–81.

68. C. Marsh, *Prescription for Energy* (London: Thorsons, 1964).

69. M. Jackson, and D. Bruck, "Sleep Abnormalities in Chronic Fatigue Syndrome/Myalgic Encephalomyelitis: A Review," *Journal of Clinical Sleep Medicine* 8, no. 6 (2012): 719–28.

70. M. Jackson, and D. Bruck, "Sleep Abnormalities in Chronic Fatigue Syndrome/Myalgic Encephalomyelitis: A Review," *Journal of Clinical Sleep Medicine* 8, no. 6 (2012): 719–28.

11. PHARMACOLOGICAL APPROACHES TO CHRONIC FATIGUE SYNDROME

1. A. Fernández, A. Perez Martin, M. Izquierdo-Martínez, M. Arruti Bustillo, F. Hernández, J. Labrado, R. Díaz-Delgado Peñas, E. Gutiérrez Rivas, C.

Palacín Delgado, J. Rivera, J. Giménez, "Chronic Fatigue Syndrome: Aetiology, Diagnosis and Treatment," *BMC Psychiatry* 9, Suppl. 1 (2009): S1.

2. K. Stange, "Healing Perceptions and Relationships," *Annals of Family Medicine* 6, no. 5 (2008): 466–68.

3. L. Dall, J. Stanford, and J. Hurst, eds., *Clinical Methods: The History, Physical, and Laboratory Examinations*, 3rd ed. (Boston: Butterworths, 1990).

4. G. Morris and M. Maes, "Oxidative and Nitrosative Stress and Immune-inflammatory Pathways in Patients with Myalgic Encephalomyelitis (ME)/Chronic Fatigue Syndrome (CFS)," *Current Neuropharmacology* 12, no. 2 (2014): 168–85.

5. C. Sostres, C. Gargallo, M. Arroyo, and A. Lanas, "Adverse Effects of Non-steroidal Anti-inflammatory Drugs (NSAIDs, Aspirin and Coxibs) on Upper Gastrointestinal Tract," *Best Practice & Research Clinical Gastroenterology* 24, no. 2 (2010): 121–32.

6. A. Kumar, R. Garg, V. Gaur, and P. Kumar, "Nitric Oxide Modulation in Protective Role of Antidepressants against Chronic Fatigue Syndrome in Mice," *Indian Journal of Pharmacology* 43, no. 3 (2011): 324–29.

7. A. Kumar, R. Garg, V. Gaur, and P. Kumar, "Nitric Oxide Modulation in Protective Role of Antidepressants against Chronic Fatigue Syndrome in Mice," *Indian Journal of Pharmacology* 43, no. 3 (2011): 324–29.

8. A. Cooper, V. Tucker, and G. Papakostas, "Resolution of Sleepiness and Fatigue: A Comparison of Bupropion and Selective Serotonin Reuptake Inhibitors in Subjects with Major Depressive Disorder Achieving Remission at Doses Approved in the European Union," *Journal of Psychopharmacology* 28, no. 2 (2014): 118–24.

9. S. Lynch, R. Seth, and S. Montgomery, "Antidepressant Therapy in the Chronic Fatigue Syndrome," *British Journal of General Practice* 41, no. 349 (1991): 339–42.

10. C. Gualtieri and L. Johnson, "Antidepressant Side Effects in Children and Adolescents," *Journal of Child and Adolescent Psychopharmacology* 16, nos. 1–2 (2006): 147–57.

11. W. Shiel, "Chronic Fatigue Syndrome: Medical Treatment," accessed July 24, 2014, www.emedicinehealth.com.

12. R. Awad, D. Levac, P. Cybulska, Z. Merali, V. Trudeau, and J. Arnason, "Effects of Traditionally Used Anxiolytic Botanicals on Enzymes of the Gamma-aminobutyric Acid (GABA) System," *Canadian Journal of Physiology and Pharmacology* 85, no. 9 (2007): 933–42.

13. D. Helton, J. Tizzano, J. Monn, D. Schoepp, and M. Kallman, "Anxiolytic and Side-effect Profile of LY354740: A Potent, Highly Selective, Orally Active Agonist for Group II Metabotropic Glutamate Receptors," *Journal of Pharmacology and Experimental Therapeutics* 284, no. 2 (1998): 651–60.

14. Z. Gotts, V. Deary, J. Newton, D. Van der Dussen, P. De Roy, and J. Ellis, "Are There Sleep-specific Phenotypes in Patients with Chronic Fatigue Syndrome? A Cross-sectional Polysomnography Analysis?" *BMJ Open* 3, no. 6 (2013): e002999.

15. A. Doble, "New Insights into the Mechanism of Action of Hypnotics," *Journal of Psychopharmacology* 13, no. 4, Suppl. 1 (1999): S11–20.

16. W. Kelly, M. Ambrose, E. Gallen, A. Houska, M. Devlin, M. Anello, R. Doyle, S. Cammon, C. Damico, L. Neri, and K. Zalewski, *Nursing Drug Handbook*, 23rd ed. (New York: Lippincott Williams and Wilkins, 2003): 14–1240.

17. R. Suhadolnik, N. Reichenbach, P. Hitzges, R. Sobol, D. Peterson, B. Henry, D. Ablashi, W. Müller, J. Schröder, and W. Carter, "Upregulation of the 2-5A Synthetase/RNase L Antiviral Pathway Associated with Chronic Fatigue Syndrome," *Clinical Infectious Diseases* 18, Suppl. 1 (1994): S96–104.

18. R. Suhadolnik, N. Reichenbach, P. Hitzges, R. Sobol, D. Peterson, B. Henry, D. Ablashi, W. Müller, J. Schröder, and W. Carter, "Upregulation of the 2-5A Synthetase/RNase L Antiviral Pathway Associated with Chronic Fatigue Syndrome," *Clinical Infectious Diseases* 18, Suppl. 1 (1994): S96–104.

19. R. Suhadolnik, N. Reichenbach, P. Hitzges, R. Sobol, D. Peterson, B. Henry, D. Ablashi, W. Müller, J. Schröder, and W. Carter, "Upregulation of the 2-5A Synthetase/RNase L Antiviral Pathway Associated with Chronic Fatigue Syndrome," *Clinical Infectious Diseases* 18, Suppl. 1 (1994): S96–104.

20. R. Razonable, "Antiviral Drugs for Viruses Other Than Human Immunodeficiency Virus," *Mayo Clinic Proceedings* 86, no. 10 (2011): 1009–26.

21. E. Iwakami, Y. Arashima, K. Kato, T. Komiya, Y. Matsukawa, T. Ikeda, Y. Arakawa, and S. Oshida, "Treatment of Chronic Fatigue Syndrome with Antibiotics: Pilot Study Assessing the Involvement of Coxiella Burnetii Infection," *Internal Medicine* 44, no. 12 (2005): 1258–63.

22. R. Hancock, "Mechanisms of Action of Newer Antibiotics for Gram-positive Pathogens," *The Lancet Infectious Diseases* 5, no. 4 (2005): 209–18.

23. P. Rishi, S. Preet, and P. Kaur, "Effect of L. Plantarum Cell-free Extract and Co-trimoxazole against Salmonella Typhimurium: A Possible Adjunct Therapy," *Annals of Clinical Microbiology and Antimicrobials* 10 (2011): 9.

24. D. Dunwell, "ME/CFS and Blastocystis Spp or Dientamoeba Fragilis: An In-house Comparison," *British Journal of General Practice* 63, no. 607 (2013): 73–74.

25. S. Parija and K. Khairnar, "Detection of Excretory Entamoeba Histolytica DNA in the Urine, and Detection of E. Histolytica DNA and Lectin Antigen in the Liver Abscess Pus for the Diagnosis of Amoebic Liver Abscess," *BMC Microbiology* 7 (2007): 41.

26. I. Esfandiarpour, S. Farajzadeh, Z. Rahnama, E. Fathabadi, and A. Heshmatkhah, "Adverse Effects of Intralesional Meglumine Antimoniate and

Its Influence on Clinical Laboratory Parameters in the Treatment of Cutaneous Leishmaniasis," *International Journal of Dermatology* 51, no. 10 (2012): 1221–25.

27. I. Esfandiarpour, S. Farajzadeh, Z. Rahnama, E. Fathabadi, and A. Heshmatkhah, "Adverse Effects of Intralesional Meglumine Antimoniate and Its Influence on Clinical Laboratory Parameters in the Treatment of Cutaneous Leishmaniasis," *International Journal of Dermatology* 51, no. 10 (2012): 1221–25.

28. M. Kiebala and S. Maggirwar, "Ibudilast, a Pharmacologic Phosphodiesterase Inhibitor, Prevents Human Immunodeficiency Virus-1 Tat-mediated Activation of Microglial Cells," *PLOS One* 6, no. 4 (2011): e18633.

29. M. Kiebala and S. Maggirwar, "Ibudilast, a Pharmacologic Phosphodiesterase Inhibitor, Prevents Human Immunodeficiency Virus-1 Tat-mediated Activation of Microglial Cells," *PLOS One* 6, no. 4 (2011): e18633.

30. D. Strayer, W. Carter, B. Stouch, S. Stevens, L. Bateman, P. Cimoch, C. Lapp, D. Peterson, and W. Mitchell, "A Double-blind, Placebo-controlled, Randomized, Clinical Trial of the TLR-3 Agonist Rintatolimod in Severe Cases of Chronic Fatigue Syndrome," *PLOS One* 7, no. 3 (2012): e31334.

31. D. See and J. Tilles, "Alpha-interferon Treatment of Patients with Chronic Fatigue Syndrome," *Immunological Investigations* 25, nos. 1–2 (1996): 153–64.

32. A. Kavelaars, W. Kuis, L. Knook, G. Sinnema, and C. Heijnen, "Disturbed Neuroendocrine-immune Interactions in Chronic Fatigue Syndrome," *The Journal of Clinical Endocrinology & Metabolism* 85, no. 2 (2000): 692–96.

33. J. Smith, E. Fritz, J. Kerr, A. Cleare, S. Wessely, and D. Mattey, "Association of Chronic Fatigue Syndrome with Human Leucocyte Antigen Class II Alleles," *Journal of Clinical Pathology* 58, no. 8 (2005): 860–63.

34. O. Fluge and O. Mella, "Clinical Impact of B-cell Depletion with the Anti-CD20 Antibody Rituximab in Chronic Fatigue Syndrome: A Preliminary Case Series," *BMC Neurology* 9 (2009): 28.

35. S. Smelter, B. Bare, *Medical Surgical Nursing: Volume 1 and 2* (New York: Lippincott Williams and Wilkins, 2004) 124–211.

36. T. Chaudhry, P. Hissaria, M. Wiese, R. Heddle, F. Kette, and W. Smith, "Oral Drug Challenges in Non-steroidal Anti-inflammatory Drug-induced Urticaria, Angioedema and Anaphylaxis," *Journal of Internal Medicine* 42, no. 6 (2012): 665–71.

37. T. Chaudhry, P. Hissaria, M. Wiese, R. Heddle, F. Kette, and W. Smith, "Oral Drug Challenges in Non-steroidal Anti-inflammatory Drug-induced Urticaria, Angioedema and Anaphylaxis," *Journal of Internal Medicine* 42, no. 6 (2012): 665–71.

38. A. Grieco, A. Forgione, L. Miele, V. Vero, A. Greco, A. Gasbarrini, and G. Gasbarrini, "Fatty Liver and Drugs," *European Review for Medical and Pharmacological Sciences* 9, no. 5 (2005): 261–63.

39. T. Mathew, "Drug-induced Renal Disease," *Medical Journal of Australia* 156, no. 10 (1992): 724–28.

40. D. Venes, C. Thomas, E. Egan, N. Morelli, and A. Nell, *Taber's Cyclopedic Medical Dictionary* 19th ed. (Philadelphia: F.A. Davis Company, 2001): 333–1229.

41. A. Cleare, E. Heap, G. Malhi, S. Wessely, V. O'Keane, and J. Miell, "Low Dose Hydrocortisone in Chronic Fatigue Syndrome: A Randomised Crossover Trial," *Lancet* 353, no. 9151 (1999): 455–58.

42. A. Wilson, I. Hickie, A. Lloyd, and D. Wakefield, "The Treatment of Chronic Fatigue Syndrome: Science and Speculation," *The American Journal of Medicine* 96, no. 6 (1994): 544–50.

43. L. Arnold, P. Keck Jr., and J. Welge, "Antidepressant Treatment of Fibromyalgia: A Meta-analysis and Review," *Psychosomatics* 41, no. 2 (2000): 104–13.

44. B. Kozier, G. Erb, and K. Blais, *Fundamentals of Nursing: Concepts, Process and Practice* (Singapore: Pearson Education Asia, 2001): 352–460.

12. ADDRESSING THE MIND

1. E. Attree, M. Arroll, C. Dancey, C. Griffith, and A. Bansal, "Psychosocial Factors Involved in Memory and Cognitive Failures in People with Myalgic Encephalomyelitis/Chronic Fatigue Syndrome," *Psychology Research and Behavior Management* 7 (2014): 72.

2. A. Baddeley, ed., *Human Memory: Theory and Practice* (Hove, UK: Psychology Press 1997).

3. B. Carruthers, A. Jain, K. De Meirleir, D. Peterson, N. Klimas, and A. Lerner, "Myalgic Encephalomyelitis/Chronic Fatigue Syndrome: Clinical Working Case Definition, Diagnostics, and Treatment Protocols," *Journal of Chronic Fatigue Syndrome* 11, no. 1 (2003): 7–36.

4. J. Findley, R. Kerns, L. Weinberg, and R. Rosenberg, "Self-efficacy As a Psychological Moderator of Chronic Fatigue Syndrome," *Journal of Behavioral Medicine* 21, no. 4 (1998): 351–62.

5. F. Friedberg and L. Jason, *Understanding Chronic Fatigue Syndrome: An Empirical Guide to Assessment and Treatment* (Washington, DC: American Psychological Association, 1998).

6. L. Jason, E. Witter, and S. Torres-Harding, "Chronic Fatigue Syndrome, Coping, Optimism and Social Support," *Journal of Mental Health* 12, no. 2 (2003): 109–18.

7. B. Marcel, A. Komaroff, L. Faioli, R. Kornish, and M. Albert, "Cognitive Deficits in Patients with CFS," *Biological Psychiatry* 40 (1996): 535–41.

8. M. Mayer, "The Role of Severe Life Stress, Social Support and Attachment in the Onset of Chronic Fatigue Syndrome," *Dissertation Abstracts International*, 60 (2000): 3605.

9. M. Mayer, "The Role of Severe Life Stress, Social Support and Attachment in the Onset of Chronic Fatigue Syndrome," *Dissertation Abstracts International*, 60 (2000): 3605.

10. M. McDaniel and G. Einstein, *Prospective Memory: An Overview and Synthesis of an Emerging Field* (New York: Sage Publications, 2007).

11. A. Missen, W. Hollingworth, N. Eaton, and E. Crawley, "The Financial and Psychological Impacts on Mothers of Children with Chronic Fatigue Syndrome (CFS/ME)," *Child: Care, Health and Development* 38, no. 4 (2012): 505–12; J. Ormrod, *Educational Psychology: Developing Learners*, 5th ed. (Upper Saddle River, NJ: Pearson/Merrill Prentice Hall, 2006).

12. D. Pountney, "Identifying and Managing Chronic Fatigue Syndrome," *British Journal of Neuroscience Nursing* 5, no. 10 (2013): 460–62.

13. D. Pountney, "Identifying and Managing Chronic Fatigue Syndrome," *British Journal of Neuroscience Nursing* 5, no. 10 (2013): 460–62.

14. S. Van Damme, G. Crombez, B. Van Houdenhove, A. Mariman, and W. Michielsen, "Well-being in Patients with Chronic Fatigue Syndrome: The Role of Acceptance," *Journal of Psychosomatic Research* 61, no. 5 (2006): 595–99.

15. S. Van Damme, G. Crombez, B. Van Houdenhove, A. Mariman, and W. Michielsen, "Well-being in Patients with Chronic Fatigue Syndrome: The Role of Acceptance," *Journal of Psychosomatic Research* 61, no. 5 (2006): 595–99.

16. S. Van Damme, G. Crombez, B. Van Houdenhove, A. Mariman, and W. Michielsen, "Well-being in Patients with Chronic Fatigue Syndrome: The Role of Acceptance," *Journal of Psychosomatic Research* 61, no. 5 (2006): 595–99.

17. N. Ware, "Toward a Model of Social Course in Chronic Illness: The Example of Chronic Fatigue Syndrome," *Culture, Medicine, and Psychiatry* 23, no. 3 (1999): 303–31.

18. N. Ware, "Toward a Model of Social Course in Chronic Illness: The Example of Chronic Fatigue Syndrome," *Culture, Medicine, and Psychiatry* 23, no. 3 (1999): 303–31.

19. N. Ware, "Toward a Model of Social Course in Chronic Illness: The Example of Chronic Fatigue Syndrome," *Culture, Medicine, and Psychiatry* 23, no. 3 (1999): 303–31.

20. B. Saltzstein, G. Wyshak, J. Hubbuch, and J. Perry, "A Naturalistic Study of the Chronic Fatigue Syndrome among Women in Primary Care," *General Hospital Psychiatry* 20, no. 5 (1998): 307–16.

21. B. Saltzstein, G. Wyshak, J. Hubbuch, and J. Perry, "A Naturalistic Study of the Chronic Fatigue Syndrome among Women in Primary Care," *General Hospital Psychiatry* 20, no. 5 (1998): 307–16.

22. B. Saltzstein, G. Wyshak, J. Hubbuch, and J. Perry, "A Naturalistic Study of the Chronic Fatigue Syndrome among Women in Primary Care," *General Hospital Psychiatry* 20, no. 5 (1998): 307–16.

23. R. Taylor, F. Friedberg, and L. Jason, *A Clinician's Guide to Controversial Illnesses: Chronic Fatigue Syndrome, Fibromyalgia and Multiple Chemical Sensitivities* (Sarasota, FL: Professional Resource Press, 2001).

24. H. Kang, B. Natelson, C. Mahan, K. Lee, and F. Murphy, "Post-traumatic Stress Disorder and Chronic Fatigue Syndrome-like Illness among Gulf War Veterans: A Population-Based Survey of 30,000 Veterans," *American Journal of Epidemiology* 157, no. 2 (2003): 141–48.

25. H. Kang, B. Natelson, C. Mahan, K. Lee, and F. Murphy, "Post-traumatic Stress Disorder and Chronic Fatigue Syndrome-like Illness among Gulf War Veterans: A Population-based Survey of 30,000 Veterans," *American Journal of Epidemiology* 157, no. 2 (2003): 141–48.

26. H. Kang, B. Natelson, C. Mahan, K. Lee, and F. Murphy, "Post-traumatic Stress Disorder and Chronic Fatigue Syndrome-like Illness among Gulf War Veterans: A Population-based Survey of 30,000 Veterans," *American Journal of Epidemiology* 157, no. 2 (2003): 141–48.

27. C. Brodsky, "Depression and Chronic Fatigue in the Workplace: Workers' Compensation and Occupational Issues," *Primary Care* 18, no. 2 (1991): 381–96.

28. T. Sampalli, E. Berlasso, R. Fox, and M. Petter, "A Controlled Study of the Effect of a Mindfulness-based Stress Reduction Technique in Women with Multiple Chemical Sensitivity, Chronic Fatigue Syndrome, and Fibromyalgia," *Journal of Multidisciplinary Healthcare* 2 (2009): 53–59.

13. COLLECTIVE EFFORTS

1. A. Lloyd and H. Pender, "The Economic Impact of Chronic Fatigue Syndrome," *Medical Journal of Australia* 157, no. 9 (1992): 599–601.

2. I. Gibson, "A New Look at Chronic Fatigue Syndrome/Myalgic Encephalomyelitis," *Journal of Clinical Pathology* 60, no. 2 (2007): 120–21.

3. I. Lewis, J. Pairman, G. Spickett, and J. Newton, "Clinical Characteristics of a Novel Subgroup of Chronic Fatigue Syndrome Patients with Postural

Orthostatic Tachycardia Syndrome," *Journal of Intern Medicine* 273, no. 5 (2013): 501–10.

4. E. Del Fabbro, S. Dalal, and E. Bruera, "Symptom Control in Palliative Care—Part II: Cachexia/Anorexia and Fatigue," *Journal of Palliative Medicine* 9, no. 2 (2006): 409–21.

5. P. Santamarina-Perez, F. Eiroa-Orosa, V. Freniche, A. Moreno-Mayos, J. Alegre, N. Saez, and C. Jacas, "Length of Disorder Does Not Predict Cognitive Dysfunction in Chronic Fatigue Syndrome," *Applied Neuropsychology* 18, no. 3 (2011): 216–22.

6. M. Meeus, I. van Eupen, E. van Baarle, V. De Boeck, A. Luyckx, D. Kos, and J. Nijs, "Symptom Fluctuations and Daily Physical Activity in Patients with Chronic Fatigue Syndrome: A Case-control Study," *Archives of Physical Medicine and Rehabilitation* 92, no. 11 (2011): 1820–26.

7. C. King and L. Jason, "Improving the Diagnostic Criteria and Procedures for Chronic Fatigue Syndrome," *Biological Psychology* 68, no. 2 (2005): 87–106.

8. N. Janssen, I. Kant, G. Swaen, P. Janssen, and C. Schröer, "Fatigue As a Predictor of Sickness Absence: Results from the Maastricht Cohort Study on Fatigue at Work," *Occupational and Environmental Medicine* 60, Suppl. 1 (2003): i71-6.

9. E. Berndt, J. Bailit, M. Keller, J. Verner, and S. Finkelstein, "Health Care Use and At-work Productivity among Employees with Mental Disorders," *Health Affairs* 19, no. 4 (2000): 244–56.

10. R. Bennett, J. Jones, D. Turk, I. Russell, and L. Matallana, "An Internet Survey of 2,596 People with Fibromyalgia," *BioMedCentral (BMC) Musculoskeletal Disorders* 8 (2007): 27.

11. "National Fibromyalgia Research Association" accessed July 23, 2014, www.nfra.net.

12. The International Association for CFS/ME, "Presidential Letter," accessed July 23, 2014, www.iacfsme.org.

13. "Introduction to HHV-6," accessed June 25, 2014, www.hhv-6foundation.org.

14. "About NICE," Accessed June 29, 2014, www.nice.org.uk.

15. "Mission and Vision," accessed May 21, 2014, www.pandoraorg.net.

16. "About Us," accessed May 23, 2014, www.rmcfa.org.

17. "About Us," accessed June 12, 2014, www.wicfs-me.org.

18. L. Jason, J. Ferrari, R. Taylor, S. Slavich, and C. Stenzel, "A National Assessment of the Service, Support, and Housing Preferences by Persons with Chronic Fatigue Syndrome: Toward a Comprehensive Rehabilitation Program," *Evaluation & the Health Professions* 19, no. 2 (1996): 194–207.

19. J. Taylor, A. Gilbertson, W. Semchuk, and J. Johnson, "Effect of Verbal Encouragement on Patient Question-asking Behaviour during Medication Counselling Support Groups," *International Journal of Pharmacy Practice* 9, no. 4 (2001): 253–59.

20. J. Trabal, P. Leyes, J. Fernández-Solá, M. Forga, and J. Fernández-Huerta, "Patterns of Food Avoidance in Chronic Fatigue Syndrome: Is There a Case for Dietary Recommendations?" *Nutrición Hospitalaria* 27, no. 2 (2012): 659–62.

21. K. Phillips, L. Faul, B. Small, P. Jacobsen, S. Apte, and H. Jim, "Comparing the Retrospective Reports of Fatigue Using the Fatigue Symptom Index with Daily Diary Ratings in Women Receiving Chemotherapy for Gynecologic Cancer," *Journal of Pain and Symptom Management* 46, no. 2 (2013): 282–88.

22. J. Chan, R. Ho, C. Wang, L. Yuen, J. Sham, and C. Chan, "Effects of Qigong Exercise on Fatigue, Anxiety, and Depressive Symptoms of Patients with Chronic Fatigue Syndrome–like Disorder: A Randomized Controlled Trial," *Evidence Based Complementary and Alternative Medicine* (2013): 485341.

23. G. Richardson, D. Epstein, C. Chew-Graham, C. Dowrick, R. Bentall, R. Morriss, S. Peters, L. Riste, K. Lovell, G. Dunn, A. Wearden, "Cost-effectiveness of Supported Self-management for CFS/ME Patients in Primary Care," *BMC Family Practice* 14 (2013): 12.

24. S. Kreijkamp-Kaspers, E. Brenu, S. Marshall, D. Staines, and M. Van Driel, "Treating Chronic Fatigue Syndrome: A Study into the Scientific Evidence for Pharmacological Treatments," *Australian Family Physician* 40, no. 11 (2011): 907–12.

25. S. Chafin, N. Christenfeld, and W. Gerin, "Improving Cardiovascular Recovery from Stress with Brief Poststress Exercise," *Health Psychology* 27, Suppl. 1 (2008): S64–72.

26. K. McCully, B. Clark, J. Kent, J. Wilson, and B. Chance, "Biochemical Adaptations to Training: Implications for Resisting Muscle Fatigue," *Canadian Journal of Physiology and Pharmacology* 69, no. 2 (1991): 274–78.

27. T. Sampalli, E. Berlasso, R. Fox, and M. Petter, "A Controlled Study of the Effect of a Mindfulness-based Stress Reduction Technique in Women with Multiple Chemical Sensitivity, Chronic Fatigue Syndrome, and Fibromyalgia," *Journal of Multidisciplinary Healthcare* 2 (2009): 53–59.

28. T. Kahlon, M. Chiu, and M. Chapman, "Steam Cooking Significantly Improves in Vitro Bile Acid Binding of Collard Greens, Kale, Mustard Greens, Broccoli, Green Bell Pepper, and Cabbage," *Nutrition Research* 28, no. 6 (2008): 351–57.

14. CONCLUSION

1. The ME Association, "Fatigue Research Symposium," accessed May 13, 2014, www.meassociation.org.uk/research/fatigue-research-symposium.

2. Centers for Disease Control and Prevention, "Diagnosing CFS," accessed May 13, 2014, www.cdc.gov/cfs/diagnosis/index.html.

3. Massachusetts CFIDS/ME and FM Association, "What Is CFIDS/ME?" accessed May 15, 2014, www.masscfids.org/about-cfidsme.

4. Centers for Disease Control and Prevention, "CFS Case Definition," accessed May 13, 2014, www.cdc.gov/cfs/case-definition/index.html.

5. J. Wilson, "20 Things People over 20 Should Stop Doing," accessed May 13, 2014, www.jarridwilson.com/20-things-people-over-20-should-stop-doing.

6. Solving ME/CFS Initiative, "Fundraising," accessed May 15, 2014, www.solvecfs.org/get-involved/fundraising.

7. Action for ME, "International Information," accessed May 15, 2014, www.actionforme.org.uk/get-informed/international-information.

8. M. Ruiz, "Risks of Self-medication Practices," *Current Drug Safety* 5, no. 4 (2010): 315–23.

9. M. Ruiz, "Risks of Self-medication Practices," *Current Drug Safety* 5, no. 4 (2010): 315–23.

10. D. Payne, "The Importance of Prevention in Health Care," *Canadian Family Physician* 47 (2001): 2211–13.

11. Massachusetts CFIDS/ME and FM Association, "Treatment," accessed May 15, 2014, www.masscfids.org/treatment.

12. M. Reyes, R. Nisenbaum, D. Hoaglin, E. Unger, C. Emmons, B. Randall, J. Stewart, S. Abbey, J. Jones, N. Gantz, S. Minden, and W. Reeves, "Prevalence and Incidence of Chronic Fatigue Syndrome in Wichita, Kansas," *Archives of Internal Medicine* 163, no. 13 (2003): 1530–36.

13. J. Stevens and D. Stephens, "Patience," *Current Biology* 18, no. 1 (2008): R11-2.

14. H. Lewine, "When Exercise Makes You Feel Worse," accessed May 13, 2014, www.intelihealth.com/print-article/chronic-fatigue-syndrome-when-exercise-makes-you-feel-worse.

15. K. Kirk, "Confidence As a Factor in Chronic Illness Care," *Journal of Advanced Nursing* 17, no. 10 (1992): 1238–42.

BIBLIOGRAPHY

PREFACE

Bagnall, A. M., P. Whiting, R. Richardson, and A. J. Sowden. "Interventions for the Treatment and Management of Chronic Fatigue Syndrome/Myalgic Encephalomyelitis." *Quality & Safety in Health Care* 11, no. 3 (2002): 284–88.

Capuron, L., L. Welberg, C. Heim, D. Wagner, L. Solomon, D. Papanicolaou, R. Craddock, Miller, A., and W. Reeves. "Cognitive Dysfunction Relates to Subjective Report of Mental Fatigue in Patients with Chronic Fatigue Syndrome." *Neuropsychopharmacology* 31, no. 8 (2006): 1777–84.

Whiting, P., A. M. Bagnall, A. J. Sowden, J. E. Cornell, C. D. Mulrow, and G. Ramírez. "Interventions for the Treatment and Management of Chronic Fatigue Syndrome: A Systematic Review." *Journal of the American Medical Association* 286, no. 11 (2001): 1360–68.

CHAPTER I

Aldrich, T. K. "Transmission Fatigue of the Rabbit Diaphragm." *Respiration Physiology* 69, no. 3 (1987): 307–19.

Heymsfield, S. B., D. Thomas, A. Bosy-Westphal, W. Shen, C. M. Peterson, and M. J. Müller. "Evolving Concepts on Adjusting Human Resting Energy Expenditure Measurements for Body Size." *Obesity Reviews* 13, no. 11 (2012): 1001–14.

Kaminski, M. V. "A New Look at Chronic Fatigue Syndrome: The Link between Antibiotics, the Intestine and Mitochondrial Dysfunction." *Mature Medicine Canada* 3 (2000): 85–89.

Meier, U., and A. M. Gressner. "Endocrine Regulation of Energy Metabolism: Review of Pathobiochemical and Clinical Chemical Aspects of Leptin, Ghrelin, Adiponectin, and Resistin." *Clinical Chemistry* 50, no. 9 (2004): 1511–25.

Rathmacher, J. A., J. C. Fuller Jr., S. M. Baier, N. N. Abumrad, H. F. Angus, and R. L. Sharp. "Adenosine-5'-Triphosphate (ATP) Supplementation Improves Low Peak Muscle Torque and Torque Fatigue during Repeated High Intensity Exercise Sets." *Journal of the International Society of Sports Nutrition* 9, no. 9 (2012): 48.

CHAPTER 2

Anderson, V. R., L. A. Jason, and L. E. Hlavaty. "A Qualitative Natural History Study of ME/CFS in the Community." *Health Care for Women International* 35, no. 1 (2014): 3–26.

Harvey, S. B., S. Wessely, D. Kuh, and M. Hotopf. "The Relationship between Fatigue and Psychiatric Disorders: Evidence for the Concept of Neurasthenia." *Journal of Psychosomatic Research* 66, no. 5 (2009): 445–54.

Porter, N., A. Lerch, L. A. Jason, M. Sorenson, M. A. Fletcher, and J. Herrington. "A Comparison of Immune Functionality in Viral versus Non-viral CFS Subtypes." *Behavioral Neuroscience* 8, no. 2 (2010): 1–8.

Tersteeg, I. M., F. S. Koopman, J. M. Stolwijk-Swüste, A. Beelen, and F. Nollet. "A 5-year Longitudinal Study of Fatigue in Patients with Late-onset Sequelae of Poliomyelitis." *Archives of Physical Medicine and Rehabilitation* 92, no. 6 (2011): 899–904.

Wookey, C. Review of *Post-viral Fatigue Syndrome: The Saga of Royal Free Disease*, by A. M. Ramsay. *The Journal of the Royal College of General Practitioners* 37, no. 305 (1987): 565.

CHAPTER 3

Hampton, T. "Researchers Find Genetic Clues to Chronic Fatigue Syndrome." *Journal of the American Medical Association* 295, no. 21 (2006): 2466–67.

Scott, L. V., S. Medbak, and T. G. Dinan. "Blunted Adrenocorticotropin and Cortisol Responses to Corticotropin-releasing Hormone Stimulation in Chronic Fatigue Syndrome." *Acta Psychiatrica Scandinavica* 97, no. 6 (1998): 450–57.

Taillefer, S. S., L. J. Kirmayer, J. M. Robbins, and J. C. Lasry. "Psychological Correlates of Functional Status in Chronic Fatigue Syndrome." *Journal of Psychosomatic Research* 53, no. 6 (2002): 1097–106.

Tersteeg, I. M., F. S. Koopman, J. M. Stolwijk-Swüste, A. Beelen, and F. Nollet. "A 5-year Longitudinal Study of Fatigue in Patients with Late-onset Sequelae of Poliomyelitis." *Archives of Physical Medicine and Rehabilitation* 92, no. 6 (2011): 899–904.

CHAPTER 4

Hardcastle, S. L., E. Brenu, S. Johnston, T. Nguyen, T. Huth, M. Kaur, S. Ramos, A. Salajegheh, D. Staines, and S. Marshall-Gradisnik. "Analysis of the Relationship between Immune Dysfunction and Symptom Severity in Patients with Chronic Fatigue Syndrome/Myalgic Encephalomyelitis (CFS/ME)." *Journal of Clinical & Cellular Immunology* 5, no. 190 (2014): 4172.

Harrower, T. P., L. J. Findley, G. Lennox, and D. G. O'Donovan. "Pathological Findings in a Case of Severe Chronic Fatigue Syndrome." *Journal of the Neurological Sciences* 238 (2005): S512–S512.

Holmes, G. P., J. E. Kaplan, N. M. Gantz, A. L. Komaroff, L. B. Schonberger, S. E. Straus, J. F. Jones, R. E. Dubois, C. Cunningham-Rundles, and S. Pahwa. "Chronic Fatigue Syndrome: A Working Case Definition." *Annals of Internal Medicine* 108, no. 3 (1988): 387–89.

Jason, L. A., S. R. Torres-Harding, A. W. Carrico, and R. R. Taylor. "Symptom Occurrence in Persons with Chronic Fatigue Syndrome." *Biological Psychology* 59, no. 1 (2002): 15–27.

Lloyd, A. R., D. Wakefield, and I. Hickie. "Immunity and the Pathophysiology of Chronic Fatigue Syndrome." *Ciba Foundation Symposium* 173 (1993): 176–92.

CHAPTER 5

Aaron, L. A., R. Herrell, S. Ashton, M. Belcourt, K. Schmaling, J. Goldberg, and D. Buchwald. "Comorbid Clinical Conditions in Chronic Fatigue." *Journal of General Internal Medicine* 16, no. 1 (2001): 24–31.

Kumae, T. "The Study for Prevention and Early Phase Detection of Chronic Fatigue by Spectral Analysis of Heart Rate. Part 2: Effects of Breeding Conditions and Exercise Stress." *Japanese Journal of Hygiene* 52 (1997): 233.

Maes, M., I. Mihaylova, M. Kubera, M. Uytterhoeven, N. Vrydags, and E. Bosmans. "Coenzyme Q10 Deficiency in Myalgic Encephalomyelitis/Chronic Fatigue Syndrome (ME/CFS) is Related to Fatigue, Autonomic and Neurocognitive Symptoms and Is Another Risk Factor Explaining the Early Mortality in ME/CFS Due to Cardiovascular Disorder." *Neuroendocrinology Letters* 30, no. 4 (2008): 470–76.

Majer, M., J. F. Jones, E. R. Unger, L. S. Youngblood, M. J. Decker, B. Gurbaxani, C. Heim, and W. C. Reeves. "Perception versus Polysomnographic Assessment of Sleep in CFS and Non-fatigued Control Subjects: Results from a Population-based Study." *BMC Neurology* 7, no. 1 (2007): 40.

Nijs, J., L. M. Paul, and K. Wallman. "Prevention of Symptom Exacerbations in Chronic Fatigue Syndrome Reply." *Journal of Rehabilitation Medicine* 40, no. 10 (2008): 884–85.

Nijs, J., M. Meeus, J. Van-Oosterwijck, K. Ickmans, I. Van-Eupen, and D. Kos. "Tired of Being Inactive: CNS Dysfunctions Explain Exercise Intolerance in Chronic Fatigue Syndrome." *Neuroscience Letters* 500 (2011): e14.

Ortega, F., and R. Zorzanelli. "Neuroimaging and the Case of Chronic Fatigue Syndrome." *Ciencia & Saude Coletiva* 16, no. 4 (2011): 2123–32.

Yancey, J. R., and S. M. Thomas. "Chronic Fatigue Syndrome: Diagnosis and Treatment." *American Family Physician* 86, no. 8 (2012): 741–46.

CHAPTER 6

Ax, S., V. H. Gregg, and D. Jones. "Chronic Fatigue Syndrome: Sufferers' Evaluation of Medical Support." *Journal of the Royal Society of Medicine* 90, no. 5 (1997): 250.

Thomas, M. A., and A. P. Smith. "Primary Healthcare Provision and Chronic Fatigue Syndrome: A Survey of Patients' and General Practitioners' Beliefs." *BMC Family Practice* 6, no. 1 (2005): 49.

Wojcik, W., A. Armstrong, and R. Kanaan. "Is Chronic Fatigue Syndrome a Neurological Condition? A Survey of UK Neurologists." *Journal of Psychosomatic Research* 70, no. 6 (2011): 573–74.

CHAPTER 7

Akagi, H., I. Klimes, and C. Bass. "Cognitive Behavioral Therapy for Chronic Fatigue Syndrome in a General Hospital—Feasible and Effective." *General Hospital Psychiatry* 23, no. 5 (2001): 254–60.

Clauson, K. A., Q. Zeng-Treitler, and S. Kandula. "Readability of Patient and Health Care Professional Targeted Dietary Supplement Leaflets Used for Diabetes and Chronic Fatigue Syndrome." *The Journal of Alternative and Complementary Medicine* 16, no. 1 (2010): 119–24.

Cox, D. L., and L. J. Findley. "The Management of Chronic Fatigue Syndrome in an Inpatient Setting: Presentation of an Approach and Perceived Outcome." *The British Journal of Occupational Therapy* 61, no. 9 (1998): 405–9.

Gilje, A. M., A. Söderlund, and K. Malterud. "Obstructions for Quality Care Experienced by Patients with Chronic Fatigue Syndrome (CFS)—A Case Study." *Patient Education and Counseling* 73, no. 1 (2008): 36–41.

Vernon, S. D., and W. C. Reeves. "The Challenge of Integrating Disparate High-content Data: Epidemiological, Clinical and Laboratory Data Collected during an In-hospital Study of Chronic Fatigue Syndrome." *Pharmacogenomics* (2006): 345–54.

Viner, R., A. Gregorowski, C. Wine, M. Bladen, D. Fisher, M. Miller, and S. El Neil. "Outpatient Rehabilitative Treatment of Chronic Fatigue Syndrome (CFS/ME)." *Archives of Disease in Childhood* 89, no. 7 (2004): 615–19.

CHAPTER 8

Dempsey, J. A., M. Amann, L. M. Romer, and J. D. Miller. "Respiratory System Determinants of Peripheral Fatigue and Endurance Performance." *Medicine and Science in Sports and Exercise* 40, no. 3 (2008): 457–61.

Freeman, R., and A. L. Komaroff. "Does the Chronic Fatigue Syndrome Involve the Autonomic Nervous System?" *The American Journal of Medicine* 102, no. 4 (1997): 357–64.

Lakhan, S. E., and A. Kirchgessner. "Gut Inflammation in Chronic Fatigue Syndrome." *Nutrition & Metabolism* 7 (2010): 79.

Vecchiet, J., F. Cipollone, K. Falasca, A. Mezzetti, E. Pizzigallo, T. Bucciarelli, S. De Laurentis, G. Affaitati, D. De Cesare, and M. A. Giamberardino. "Relationship between Musculoskeletal Symptoms and Blood Markers of Oxidative Stress in Patients with Chronic Fatigue Syndrome." *Neuroscience Letters* 335, no. 3 (2003): 151–54.

CHAPTER 9

DeLuca, J., S. K. Johnson, and B. H. Natelson. "Neuropsychiatric Status of Patients with Chronic Fatigue Syndrome: An Overview." *Toxicology and Industrial Health* 10, nos. 4–5 (1993): 513–22.

Levy, J. A. "Viral Studies of Chronic Fatigue Syndrome." *Clinical Infectious Diseases: An Official Publication of the Infectious Diseases Society of America* 18 (1994): S117–20.

Morris, G., and M. Maes. "A Neuro-immune Model of Myalgic Encephalomyelitis/Chronic Fatigue Syndrome." *Metabolic Brain Disease* 28, no. 4 (2013): 523–40.

Papanicolaou, D. A., J. D. Amsterdam, S. Levine, S. M. McCann, R. C. Moore, C. H. Newbrand, and G. Allen. "Neuroendocrine Aspects of Chronic Fatigue Syndrome." *Neuroimmunomodulation* 11, no. 2 (2004): 65–74.

CHAPTER 10

Alraek, T., M. S. Lee, T.-Y. Choi, H. Cao, and J. Liu. "Complementary and Alternative Medicine for Patients with Chronic Fatigue Syndrome: A Systematic Review." *BMC Complementary and Alternative Medicine* 11, no. 1 (2011): 87.

Christopher, G., and M. Thomas. "Social Problem Solving in Chronic Fatigue Syndrome: Preliminary Findings." *Stress and Health* 25, no. 2 (2009): 161–69.

Dykman, K. D., C. Tone, C. Ford, and R. A. Dykman. "The Effects of Nutritional Supplements on the Symptoms of Fibromyalgia and Chronic Fatigue Syndrome." *Integrative Physiological and Behavioral Science* 33, no. 1 (1998): 61–71.

Knoop, H., J. Van der Meer, and G. Bleijenberg. "Guided Self-instructions for People with Chronic Fatigue Syndrome: Randomised Controlled Trial." *The British Journal of Psychiatry* 193, no. 4 (2008): 340–41.

CHAPTER 11

Iwakami, E., Y. Arashima, K. Kato, T. Komiya, Y. Matsukawa, T. Ikeda, Y. Arakawa, and S. Oshida. "Treatment of Chronic Fatigue Syndrome with Antibiotics: Pilot Study Assessing the Involvement of Coxiella Burnetii Infection." *Internal Medicine* 44, no. 12 (2005): 1258–63.

Kreijkamp-Kaspers, S., E. W. Brenu, S. Marshall, D. Staines, and M. K. Van Driel. "Treating Chronic Fatigue Syndrome: A Study into the Scientific Evidence for Pharmacological Treatments." *Australian Family Physician* 40, no. 11 (2011): 907.

Lerner, A. M., S. Beqaj, J. T. Fitzgerald, K. Gill, C. Gill, and J. Edington. "Subset-directed Antiviral Treatment of 142 Herpesvirus Patients with Chronic Fatigue Syndrome." *Virus Adaptation and Treatment* 2 (2010): 47–57.

Snell, C. R., S. R. Stevens, and J. M. VanNess. "Chronic Fatigue Syndrome, Ampligen, and Quality of Life: A Phenomenological Perspective." *Journal of Chronic Fatigue Syndrome* 8, nos. 3–4 (2001): 117–21.

CHAPTER 12

Assefi, N. P., T. V. Coy, D. Uslan, W. R. Smith, and D. Buchwald. "Financial, Occupational, and Personal Consequences of Disability in Patients with Chronic Fatigue Syndrome and Fibromyalgia Compared to Other Fatiguing Conditions." *The Journal of Rheumatology* 30, no. 4 (2003): 804–8.

Deluca, J., C. Christodoulou, B. J. Diamond, E. D. Rosenstein, N. Kramer, and B. H. Natelson. "Working Memory Deficits in Chronic Fatigue Syndrome: Differentiating between Speed and Accuracy of Information Processing." *Journal of the International Neuropsychological Society* 10, no. 1 (2004): 101–9.

Kang, H. K., B. H. Natelson, C. M. Mahan, K. Y. Lee, and F. M. Murphy. "Post-traumatic Stress Disorder and Chronic Fatigue Syndrome-like Illness among Gulf War Veterans: A Population-based Survey of 30,000 Veterans." *American Journal of Epidemiology* 157, no. 2 (2003): 141–48.

Stone, A. A., J. E. Broderick, L. S. Porter, and L. Krupp. "Fatigue and Mood in Chronic Fatigue Syndrome Patients: Results of a Momentary Assessment Protocol Examining Fatigue and Mood Levels and Diurnal Patterns." *Annals of Behavioral Medicine* 16, no. 3 (1994): 228–34.

Ware, N. C. "Suffering and the Social Construction of Illness: The Delegitimation of Illness Experience in Chronic Fatigue Syndrome." *Medical Anthropology Quarterly* 6, no. 4 (1992): 347–61.

CHAPTER 13

Aylward, M. "Government's Expert Group Has Reached Consensus on Prognosis of Chronic Fatigue Syndrome." *British Medical Journal* 313, no. 7061 (1996): 885.

Friedberg, F., D. W. Leung, and J. Quick. "Do Support Groups Help People with Chronic Fatigue Syndrome and Fibromyalgia? A Comparison of Active and Inactive Members." *The Journal of Rheumatology* 32, no. 12 (2005): 2416–20.

Schröer, C., M. Janssen, L. Van Amelsvoort, H. Bosma, G. Swaen, F. Nijhuis, and J. Van-Eijk. "Organizational Characteristics As Predictors of Work Disability: A Prospective Study among Sick Employees of For-profit and Not-for-profit Organizations." *Journal of Occupational Rehabilitation* 15, no. 3 (2005): 435–45.

CHAPTER 14

Carballo, A. M. "On Open Door to Hope for Chronic Fatigue Syndrome." *Revista de Enfermería* 33, no. 12 (2010): 4.

Chalder, T., P. Wallace, and S. Wessely. "Self-help Treatment of Chronic Fatigue in the Community: A Randomized Controlled Trial." *British Journal of Health Psychology* 2, no. 3 (1997): 189–97.

Jason, L. A., A. Witter, and S. Torres-Harding. "Chronic Fatigue Syndrome, Coping, Optimism and Social Support." *Journal of Mental Health* 12, no. 2 (2003): 109–18.

INDEX

ABOUT THE AUTHOR

Naheed Ali, MD, PhD, began writing professionally in 2005, and he has taught at colleges where he lectured on various biomedical topics. Additional information is available online at NaheedAli.com.